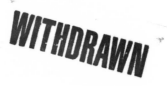

TEEN OBESITY

HOW SCHOOLS CAN BE THE NUMBER ONE SOLUTION TO THE PROBLEM

William L. Fibkins

Rowman & Littlefield Education
Lanham, Maryland • Toronto • Oxford
2006

Published in the United States of America
by Rowman & Littlefield Education
A Division of Rowman & Littlefield Publishers, Inc.
A wholly owned subsidiary of The Rowman & Littlefield Publishing Group,
Inc.
4501 Forbes Boulevard, Suite 200, Lanham, Maryland 20706
www.rowmaneducation.com

PO Box 317
Oxford
OX2 9RU, UK

British Library Cataloguing in Publication Information Available

Library of Congress Cataloging-in-Publication Data

Fibkins, William L.
  Teen obesity : how schools can be the number one solution to the problem /
William L. Fibkins.
    p. cm.
  Includes bibliographical references.
  ISBN-13: 978-1-57886-511-6 (hardcover : alk. paper)
  ISBN-10: 1-57886-511-5 (hardcover : alk. paper)
  ISBN-13: 978-1-57886-512-3 (pbk. : alk. paper)
  ISBN-10: 1-57886-512-3 (pbk. : alk. paper)
  1. Obesity in adolescence. 2. Teenagers—Nutrition. 3. Weight loss. 4.
School management and organization. I. Title.
  RJ399.C6F53 2006
  616.3'9800835—dc22   2006014301

♾™ The paper used in this publication meets the minimum requirements of
American National Standard for Information Sciences—Permanence of Paper
for Printed Library Materials, ANSI/NISO Z39.48-1992.
Manufactured in the United States of America.

To my grandchildren,
Kaitlin, Kristina, Sophia, Harry, Andrew, and Jack.

They are young children who are much loved and nourished in body and mind by caring parents. However, we all know that as children move into adolescence, they can be lured into unhealthy habits no matter how much they are loved and cared for by parents. My hope is that they, like the teenagers in this book, will have teachers in their lives who will care about their health and well-being, who will quickly intervene if they observe them heading into an unhealthy lifestyle, and who will be major sources of support for them and their parents.

CONTENTS

CONTENTS

FOREWORD

As Dr. William Fibkins, my father, suggests in this book, schools can play an important role in addressing the health and well-being issues of students and staff. As a managing chef at a school with an innovative food service program that serves healthy food and drink each day to students and staff, I am well aware that a critical part of the intervention process to keep adolescents and preadolescents healthy is preparing and presenting healthy food and drink in an attractive, stress-free dining setting where students are nourished, nurtured, and given a needed respite from their often busy school day. A place to rebuild their energy supply so they feel renewed and ready to use their minds when they return to the classroom. A place where they want to be. Another critical part of the intervention process is offering the same dining experience to staff, who also need to be nourished, be nurtured, be given a respite, and be presented with ongoing opportunities to learn how to maintain a healthy lifestyle so they can be effective role models for students.

In my experience this intervention process begins with instilling a desire on the part of the cafeteria staff to be passionate about food so students and staff can taste the care that goes into the finished product. That process requires a clear message of support from the school administration that the food service personnel are a vital and professional part of the school's mission to improve the academics, health, and well-being of every member of the school community and are an integral part of the whole school experience. Every member of the staff needs to be appreciated for what they do and be given ongoing professional development opportunities to acquire the new skills needed to prepare healthy food and drink. This educative process means moving away from a model that treats the cafeteria simply as a fast-food place where food personnel are often viewed as unimportant to a model in which food personnel are viewed as professionals with the mission of teaching students about the value of healthy food and drink and how to develop healthy habits and lifestyle. Learning about healthy eating is a lifelong tool. If you present a delicious product, students, staff, and parents will respond.

In the end the philosophy of the school regarding where, what, and how students eat matters a great deal to how they respond academically, socially, and emotionally. In my school the food served each day and the attractive, welcoming ambience of the café dining room sends a message to students and staff that their efforts are important and that the café staff appreciates their efforts by making sure they have a proper space and nurturing food. Unfortunately, many school cafeterias are dreary places, with the result that students and staff get the message that they are not appreciated and that what they eat, where they eat, and how they eat are not important.

This book is an important contribution to the current national debate on how to combat the epidemic of overweight and obese teens. The data in the book about innovative school-based programs such as the United Kingdom's Whole School Food Policy and how to implement the newly mandated Local Wellness Policies that provide a needed roadmap as to how school leaders, school wellness councils, parents, and community activists can begin rethinking the value of the school dining experience, as well as how to increase physical activity for students. Schools can play a major role in helping students avoid becoming overweight and obese and having related health and personal problems. We do know how to proceed and indeed, as this book points out, have successful models in place such as the Circle of Wellness model proposed by my father.

Brand J. Fibkins
Ross School
East Hampton, New York

1

WHY PREVENTING TEEN OBESITY SHOULD BE A PRIORITY FOR SCHOOLS

The American Heart Association reports that overweight and obesity, especially among children and teens, have emerged as serious threats to our nation's health. They have risen rapidly among women, men, and children of all racial groups. This trend is projected to continue. The frightening facts are that 16% of all children and teens in the United States are overweight.[1] According to the National Center for Health Statistics, overweight and obesity continued to increase dramatically during the late 1990s for Americans of all ethnic groups, all ages, and both genders. It is a major health problem that afflicts teens in every community, economic class, and culture. Among children and teens ages six through nineteen, 15%, almost 9 million, are overweight according to the 1999–2000 data, or triple what the proportion was in 1980. In addition, the data show that another 15% of children and teens ages six through nineteen are considered at risk of becoming overweight.[2]

Obesity can be defined as an excessive accumulation of body fat that results in individuals being at least 20% heavier than their ideal body weight. Overweight is defined as any weight in excess of the ideal range. Obesity is a common eating disorder associated with adolescence. Some teenagers are at higher risk of being overweight and obese than their peers.[3] According to the United States Department of Agriculture's Center for Nutrition Policy and Promotion, children are more at risk when either parent or both parents are overweight or obese, the children live in poverty, the family consumes a high proportion of calories from fat, and the children and parents are avid television watchers.[4]

However, according to the American Heart Association, while the obesity epidemic threatens everyone, not everyone is equally at risk. For example, among children and adolescents, obesity is more common among African Americans and Hispanics; the highest regional prevalence of obesity is consistently in the South; lower incomes are associated with higher prevalence of obesity; people in some communities have limited opportunities to make healthy food choices; and lack of physical activity, a major risk factor for obesity, is notably high among African American and Hispanic children and adolescents. The Centers for Disease Control and Prevention (CDC) also points out that physical inactivity and unhealthy eating are two primary causes of obesity and are responsible for at least 300,000 preventable deaths each year. The cost of diseases associated with obesity has been estimated at almost 100 billion dollars per year.[5] Yet according to the CDC, daily participation in high school physical education classes dropped from 42% in 1991 to 21% in 1999.[6]

There are also dramatic changes taking place in family and community life that are contributing to the rise in the number of overweight and obese teens. As Robert D. Putnam suggests, there has been an erosion of America's connectedness and community involvement over the past several decades. The century-long increase in divorce rates and the more recent increase in one-parent families have resulted in the doubling of one-parent households since 1950. The fraction of adults who are married and have children at home was sliced by more than one third from 40% in 1970 to 26% in 1997. The traditional family unit is down—a lot.

Putnam also points out that the fraction of married Americans who definitely say "our whole family eats together" has declined a third, from about 50% to 34% in just the last two decades. Putnam also suggests that the effect of electronic entertainment, above all television, on our leisure time has been substantial. Students are part of the TV generation. In addition, PTA membership nationwide plummeted from a membership high in the early 1960s of almost fifty members per one hundred families with school-age children to less than twenty members per hundred in 1997. Many parents are disengaging from their children's schooling.[7]

What we are seeing in our communities is the emergence of two-career and one-parent families, pressure on time and money, longer commutes to work, children and parents eating in different shifts, and an increase in passive TV watching. All of these issues have led to a decline in parental involvement with children's schooling and an increase in the amount of time children are on their own and at risk of developing unhealthy lifestyles such as relying on junk food and fast food while being physically inactive when watching TV. As reporter Laurie Tarkan suggests, 87% of parents say that it is "very important" or "extremely important" to eat together as a family.[8] But as parent Janette Pazer points out, "I feel guilty because it's supposed to be very important but it just doesn't work with our schedule. I'd have to leave work an hour early and try to cook while they're hanging onto me for attention and asking for homework help."[9]

The diminished time that families have to spend and eat together has serious consequences in addition to fostering poor eating habits for both children and parents that can lead to being overweight, obese, and unhealthy. As Tarkan suggests, a 2004 survey of twelve-to-seventeen-year-olds by the National Center on Addiction and Substance Abuse at Columbia University found that teenagers who reported eating two or fewer dinners a week with family members were more than one and a half times as likely to smoke, drink, or use illegal substances than were teenagers who had five to seven family dinners a week. Tarkan reports that a study from the University of Minnesota published in 2004 found that adolescent girls who reported having more frequent family meals and a positive atmosphere during those meals were less likely to have eating disorders. Yet as researcher Dr. Leann Birch suggests, what foods are available in a household may have greater impact on healthier food intake than families eating together.[10]

There is clear and persuasive evidence that obesity is a major health problem for teenagers. Dramatic shifts in family life patterns have placed the schools at the center for education and intervention. This should come as no surprise to many readers who are involved with teenagers as administrators, academic teachers, health teachers, coaches and physical education teachers, school nurses, school psychologists, and social workers. Visit any middle school, junior high school, or high school and no doubt you will observe overweight and obese students. Many are not hard to identify. There are obese students who struggle physically and emotionally to get through the day. Their excessive weight takes its toll. Just getting to school and from class to class wears them down.

And then there are the overweight students, so-called "chunky" teens who may be on the way to obesity but can still manage their daily routines. They, too, fall into the at-risk group—at risk of cardiovascular disease, high blood cholesterol, high blood pressure, type 2 diabetes, heart disease, stroke, some forms of cancer, a shortened life expectancy, and social disabilities and unhappiness that may cause stress and even mental illness unless they receive early intervention, referral to sources of help in the school and community, ongoing support, and regular monitoring as they begin to redirect their lives and become healthy and active members of the school community. They cannot be left to lead a life in which they are bullied, made targets of physical and verbal abuse, given hurtful labels such as "fatso," "pregnant," "having twins," "hippo," "two ton," "slob," or "garbage eater," and rejected and isolated by the school community. These obese and overweight teens are also vulnerable to the addictions of tobacco, alcohol, and drugs. As the reader probably knows from personal and professional experience, when you are feeling stressed and overwhelmed, the drink, pill, or cigarette—sometimes all three for some teens—does calm you and for a while softens the physical and emotional hurt you are feeling. However, the choice to turn to these addictions often results in more distress and a return to binges of unhealthy eating in hopes of finding some area of calm and well-being. In my counseling of overweight and obese teens, I have found that many of them have multiple addictions in addition to food.

We need to take action. I argue that schools are ideally placed to provide the education and intervention needed. Why? Schools are where teens can be found each day. Many bring their personal, health, and well-being problems to school each day looking for the chance to redirect their lives and become successful students. As I said earlier, many are not hard to identify. Their faces, bodies, and personalities are often characterized by the chronic fatigue and low self-esteem experienced by overweight and obese teens. Many teens can successfully hide their problems with tobacco, drugs, alcohol, physical and sexual abuse, and family violence for a while. But there is no hiding for teens who are obese or overweight. The problem is right there for everyone to see.

Therefore, I believe that educators have been presented with the opportunity to intervene with these students and put a stop to our long history of either ignoring their problems or, sadly, treating overweight and obese students as victims who are routinely targeted with abuse. I argue that schools, in fact, are ideally positioned to teach students about eating the right foods as well as modeling healthy lifestyles. Many overweight or obese teens, like all adolescents, are looking for the opportunity to redirect their lives and become healthy, successful achievers and contributing members of the school community, to fit in, to be safe, to be affirmed, to be included, to have a future, and to walk the hallways without daily facing a gauntlet of rejection, name-calling, and bullying. In my experience as a school psychologist and education reformer, I have observed that no matter how much training educators are given in preventing bullying, the hallways in our large secondary schools still belong to the students, some of whom are abusive and looking to unleash their hostility on a vulnerable target, such as an overweight or obese teen. There is no place to hide, and the only alternatives for the victim are to be absent, to be late to class, or to skip the class—alternatives that often lead to failure and dropping out.

As the American Heart Association suggests, there is an epidemic of excess. The numbers of overweight and obese teens are on the rise. The American Heart Association reports that during the 2003–2004 school year, officials in Arkansas gathered body mass index (BMI) figures on nearly 346,000 public school students from prekindergarten through twelfth grade that showed that 38% of children were either overweight (21%) or at risk for overweight (17%).[11]

As the No Child Left Behind Act suggests, our mission in the schools is to ensure that every child has what he or she needs to be safe, healthy, and cared for in order to learn.[12] In order to ensure that obese teens get what they need to be safe, healthy, and cared for in order to learn, I argue that the problem of teen obesity needs to be elevated to a priority in our school intervention systems. It must be given the same priority as other personal, health, and well-being problems among teenagers, such as tobacco use, substance abuse, physical and sexual abuse, family violence, eating disorders, bullying, and so forth.

Ensuring this kind of action requires that overweight and obese students receive early identification, intervention, referrals to sources of help in the school and community, regular monitoring of progress or lack of progress, and education and support for parents of these children, through the schools' Child Study Teams and other committees that monitor student health and achievement. Ensuring that overweight and obese teens are safe, healthy, and cared for in order to learn requires school administrators, counselors, nurses, teacher leaders, and parent advocates to send messages to staff, students, and parents that they are expected to be sources of help, education, and referrals for overweight and obese students. They cannot look the other way when they observe a student who is overweight and on the road to obesity or, far worse, engage in stereotyping and negative labeling of obese students in faculty-room dialogues or allow students to scapegoat and abuse obese peers.

Caring and respect for obese students, ensuring that every obese student has what he or she needs to be safe, healthy, and cared for in order to learn, begins with strong leadership and commitment followed by early identification and intervention. California state superintendent of instruction Jack O'Connell provides such an example by promoting strong and clear policies that link student health to academic achievement. He is taking steps to improve student health and academic success with his initiatives to combat the epidemic of childhood obesity, implement nutritional standards for school food services, promote quality instruction in health and physical education, and foster a supportive and positive school climate.

He argues that obesity needs to be given the same strong response as other teen health and well-being problems, such as tobacco, alcohol, and drug use.[13]

I believe that the challenge of effectively responding to the growing number of personal health and well-being problems that students are now bringing into our secondary schools has given the schools a great opportunity to be credible at a time when schools and teachers are often viewed as out-of-date and ineffective in helping students to be successful academic students and future citizens. As Bill Gates, founder of Microsoft, suggested at the National Education Summit on High Schools,

> America's high schools are obsolete. They were designed fifty years ago to meet the needs of another age. Until we design them to meet the needs of the 21st century, we will keep limiting, even ruining, the lives of millions of Americans every year. Those who drop out of school have it worse. Only forty percent have jobs. One in four turns to welfare or other kinds of government assistance. Everyone agrees this is tragic. But these are our high schools that keep letting kids fall through the cracks, and we act as if it can't be helped. It can be helped. We designed these schools; we can redesign them. The basic building blocks of better high schools include making sure kids have a number of adults who know them, look out for them, and push them to achieve.[14]

In my view, secondary schools face three major challenges. They have to find ways to remain relevant community institutions that, as Bill Gates suggests, can meet the needs of students in the twenty-first century, raise academic standards and student achievement, and successfully intervene to help students plagued by personal, health, and well-being problems. I believe these challenges and their solutions are all intertwined and must be addressed in a comprehensive plan. Simply put, secondary schools cannot remain relevant if they ignore students who are failing or performing poorly because of problems with tobacco, drug, and alcohol abuse, eating disorders, physical and sexual abuse, obesity, and so forth. And secondary schools cannot expect to raise student achievement levels if a portion of their student body is afflicted by personal, health, and well-being problems that are serving as roadblocks to academic achievement. Why would parents, citizens, and educators themselves support an institution that can't deliver a successful response to growing and glaring problems that have huge negative consequences for students? No, secondary schools are not the cause of these problems, but they are being challenged, prodded, and even forced to redesign to play a major role in helping teens solve these problems.

I believe California state superintendent Jack O'Connell grasped the seriousness concerning the continued relevance of secondary schools as leaders in our communities and the important link between health and well-being and academic success when he suggested that California needs to send a clear message that the state should continue to fund learning-support programs that prevent drug use or violence, provide nutrition services, and promote physical activity. Students need to be active and healthy and have a safe environment in which to learn and thrive over time in order to be successful in school. O'Connell says, "We know that alcohol, tobacco and other drug use is related to reduced attention spans, lower investment in school and homework, a more negative attitude toward school, lower motivation and increased absenteeism. Fortunately we have programs that can improve both academic and behavioral outcomes by fostering a supportive and positive school climate."[15]

The new national attention to the problem of obesity, long a problem that has not been given priority by educators, now requires that schools address obesity with the same commitment as is given to student use and abuse of alcohol, drugs, tobacco, and so forth. Obesity, like these problems, often results in a lower investment in school and homework, a more negative attitude toward school, lower motivation, and absenteeism.

Combating the epidemic of teen obesity requires, as O'Connell suggests, programs that have the potential to improve both academic and behavioral outcomes by fostering a supporting and positive school climate. I believe our school programs need to be multifaceted, involving social and emotional learning, with the major goal of helping students to be both healthy and good achievers. Overweight and obese teens not only need to learn healthy eating habits and engage in ongoing and regular physical activity, but they also need to learn how to fend off rejection, hurtful labeling, name-calling, physical and emotional abuse, and victimization. Simply put, in order to improve their self-esteem, they have to learn how to fight for their own survival and deal with peers and adults who abuse and malign them. They need social and emotional learning skills so they can fend off abuse while putting their energy into recovery.

An example of this kind of social and emotional learning, which I will expand on in later chapters, can be a support group offered by a counselor or teacher each morning before school to help obese students learn how to handle anticipated problems, how to select healthy food, and how to seek out supportive peers, teachers, and esteem-building activities. Schools can also offer support to obese students on weekends by using the Internet and telephone and by offering support groups in collaboration with community agencies. The goal of this kind of social and emotional learning is to help obese students learn how to navigate through the school day and weekends without rejection and falling into poor eating habits, knowing they have a variety of support groups to turn to.

As researchers Roberta G. Simmons and Dale A. Blyth advise, it is important to create "arenas of comfort" in schools for troubled and unhealthy students as they try to redirect their lives. Troubled students do better in terms of both their own self-esteem and behavioral coping methods if there is some area of comfort to turn to. Not surprisingly, Simmons and Blyth suggest that if a student is comfortable in some environments, life arenas, and role relationships, then discomfort in another arena can be tolerated and mastered. There needs to be some arena of life or some set of role relationships with which the student can feel relaxed and comfortable, to which he or she can withdraw and become invigorated.[16]

I believe Bill Gates is right on target when he recommends that one of the major building blocks in redesigning our high schools is making sure kids have a number of adults who know them, look out for them, and push them to achieve. Every student, including the overweight and obese, needs at least one caring adult in the school to be in his or her corner. This can be an administrator, teacher, coach, nurse, counselor, hallway monitor, or community advocate who is accessible and available and who has the skills, commitment, energy, and desire to teach obese teens the skills they need to be safe, healthy, and able to learn and achieve to their maximum potential—a confidant, cheerleader, and advisor who is able to offer support but also tough love and confrontation when a teen is slipping into bad habits.

The National Association of Secondary School Principals report *Breaking Ranks II* also envisions a dramatically different high school, much along the lines suggested by Bill Gates. This organization sees making schools more student centered with personalized programs, support services, and personalized learning where students see their learning as meaningful and relevant. Among the recommendations of the report is that every high school student have a Personal Adult Advocate to help him or her personalize the education experience and who knows the aspirations, strengths, and weaknesses of each student and is able to interact with "hard to reach" parents.[17]

In the end, if we are to be successful in redesigning our high schools and addressing the personal, health, and well-being issues of students, such as obesity, we are going to need educators who take notice of students who are unhealthy and troubled, know how to engage these students and hear their stories, know how to provide health information and guide them to the many sources of help in the school and community, offer ongoing support and an arena of comfort, engage the students' parents in seeking help with obesity issues, and coach the recovering teen into being a peer counselor/advocate for other students afflicted by obesity, with its often related problems of alcohol, drug, or tobacco abuse and poor peer relationships. An important part of this process is helping educators move beyond the statistics and data about obesity and helping them focus on what it is like to be an obese teen. They need to walk in their shoes and begin to feel how tough it is to wake up each morning knowing that a decision to go to school means you are in for one bout after another. Bad things can happen to many obese teens while they are trying to get an education.

Let's walk with Dylan, an obese tenth-grade student who attends a large suburban high school with over 2,300 students. Dylan's case represents a composite of overweight and obese teens I have counseled and observed. While it may be easy for many students to remain anonymous in a school of 2,300, obese students do not enjoy this cloak of safety. They stand out and become targets, and the daily trek to school only adds to the home problems of students like Dylan.

Dylan's parents are divorced. He hasn't seen his father in five years. His mother, Margo, who is also obese, works two jobs to, as she says, "keep us going." She works cleaning rooms at a local hotel from 11:00 a.m. to 2:00 p.m., then as a checkout person at a local supermarket from 3:00 p.m. to 7:30 p.m. Dylan says he runs the house and tries to take some of the burden off his mother by cleaning the rented apartment, doing the laundry, and putting together some kind of dinner for his brother, Kyle, and sister, Kate, which is usually pizza or takeout from a Chinese restaurant nearby.

Margo hopes this will be the last stop for a while. The family has moved three times in the past two years. She just wishes Dylan would be happier. As she says, "I pray each day that he finds some friends and nice teachers in this new school. He used to be such a smart and handsome kid. Now, with all the moving and troubles, he's gotten so fat. I feel so bad for him. But I have all I can do to just get by. He needs help, but I don't have time to go to the school. I just pray that we get by and nobody gets sick. I have no health insurance. It scares me. I am trying to get back to school to finish my high school diploma, but I have no time. I just hope the kids at this new school go easy on Dylan. They don't know all the troubles and hurt he's been through. He doesn't need any more problems. Maybe some nice teacher will take him under his wing." I believe Margo's plea can be heard in every school from overburdened parents. They are looking to the schools for some kind of a safety net for their children and themselves. It is a plea that schools can respond to.

The verbal assaults and negative self-assessments begin early in the morning for Dylan, starting as he glances in the mirror as he shaves. He talks out loud to himself, his eyes filled with tears: "What a fat shit! Look at me! Revolting! I disgust myself and everyone at school. I can see the disgust in the eyes of the kids and some teachers. I used to be thin and a happy kid. Now I have no friends, my clothes never fit right, and I am sick of wearing all those dark colors to cover my stomach. I just want to go back to bed. I wish I didn't have to go to school. But Mom will be upset if I stay home. Maybe today will be different. A better day."

But it's not a better day. The verbal ridiculing and the physical shoving and pushing from the other kids start at the bus stop and continue through the day with few letups—at the bus stop; on the bus; in homeroom; in class; in the gym, where he never undresses; and on the bus back home again. The only escape during the day is at lunchtime, when he walks alone to the nearby McDonald's to grab a burger and fries. All the other kids are busy talking about parties, college, dating, sports, music, and dances. They leave him alone. It's his time-out room, the only time he feels safe. The cigarette smoked on the way also quiets his nerves, as do the burger and fries. He takes another smoke on the walk back to school. It's his daily diet. Frozen pizza for breakfast and burgers and fries for lunch, a daily diet that includes the side dish of verbal and physical abuse. And then the diet at home, most nights Chinese and pizza takeout for dinner plus the half pack of smokes to keep him calm.

Over time, obese teens like Dylan learn how to hide. It's their only safety net and path to survival. Many learn how to feign illness, cut class, and convince their parents that it is time to drop out. Their only outlets are food and TV. The phone never rings for them except for the calls from the school bringing bad news about failing grades, class cutting, and lack of motivation, calls that bring only more burdens for the Margos of the world without the hope of solutions. For many obese teens like Dylan, it's a lonely, solitary life without much of a future. Many of these overweight and obese teens feel anxious and out of sorts. They are not well. Dylan's weight has gone up to 298 pounds on a five foot eight inch frame—298 pounds, a number unknown to him as he has no scale or regular physical checkup. And he doesn't know his blood pressure is high, 180/135 or 190/140 each day, with total cholesterol over 380 and blood sugar off the charts. Dylan thinks he is just unhappy and has landed in a bad place thanks to his father's walking out on them. But it's more than that. Dylan is on the road to serious illness. No, he is not committing suicide, but the path he is on may have the same outcome, an early death.

I believe the hurt and conflict that accompany Dylan's daily trek to school need to be felt and understood by educators so that they will be motivated to give top priority to helping obese and overweight teens and guide/teach them to find healthier lifestyles. They need to mentally walk the walk with students like Dylan, feel their isolation, and offer a helping hand. I argue that the best way to motivate educators to want to intervene with students like Dylan is to encourage them to move beyond the data about obesity. I believe numbers alone are neutral and distant and fail to call upon educators to act. Yes, educators require information and need to understand that 16% of children and teens are overweight and at risk of serious long-term illness and early death, that obesity can be defined as an excessive accumulation of body fat that results in individuals being at least 20% heavier than their ideal weight, and that obesity can lead to social disabilities and unhappiness and even mental illness.[18]

But these data lack the pain, the hurt, and the constant rejection faced by obese teens. The data don't capture what it is like for an obese teen like Dylan to be at least 20% heavier than his peers, to be socially rejected and a candidate for mental illness. The data don't capture how many obese teens like Dylan begin to believe the hurtful words coming from the name-calling and verbal abuse they experience each day. Many teens like Dylan begin to believe that they are of little worth and that no one cares about them. They begin to see themselves as kids nobody would miss or wonder about if they never returned to school, kids whom many peers and some educators would be happy to be rid of because they are "different," don't fit the "model" of the student body, and have constant problems with absenteeism, tardiness, and confrontations with other students.

Educators also need to raise awareness that they, like it or not, have become the major source of help and intervention for obesity, overweight, and related health and well-being problems. As the report about obesity by the National Center for Health Statistics says, the development of a personal identity and body image is an important goal for adolescents. The report reads, "Your parents, physicians and teachers can help you. If you think you are overweight, talk to a trusted adult about what you can do to improve your health."[19] In my research into student life and schooling, I have found that the one constant "trusted adult" for troubled teens is often a classroom teacher, coach, counselor, school nurse, assistant principal, hallway monitor, or other school employee who has decided, as the American Heart Association suggests, that "we need to take action." It's a process that often begins with a caring peer being a source of help and directing the obese student to a trusted adult who knows how to guide the student, as well as the parent(s), to the many sources of help in the school and community, not simply leaving obese and overweight students on their own at the margins of school life. As the American Heart Association suggests, attacking the obesity problem means focusing extra attention on those at greatest risk.[20]

However, I urge the reader to keep in mind that not every student with a weight issue is obese, lives in poverty, has little access to healthy food, and lacks medical support. There are many teens who hover at the edge of being overweight. They don't stand out in hallways or at the bus stop. They are described as "a little chunky," but they don't receive the slings and arrows of the noticeably obese teen. Rather, the emotional scars they receive from their weight come from being the butt of subtle, and sometimes not-so-subtle, assaults on their weight at home, often from so-called loving family members. No doubt readers have heard these verbal assaults in their personal and professional experience, such as "I am only telling you to watch your weight for your own good," or "I am only talking to you about your weight because I love you. Do you really think I want to spend my time watching your weight? I've got better things to do." I believe these kinds of comments drive many overweight teens into a cycle of "no one will love me if I don't lose weight, but I can't seem to lose weight on my own." Prodding, pushing, demanding conversations about weight can pack a powerful negative punch and drain a confused teen of self-esteem.

Here is an example of how an important family member prodded a teenager into weight loss she was not ready to do on her own. I believe author Abby Ellin's description of her grandmother's obsession with weight offers valuable insight into how conversations about weight can be hurtful to teens and make them question their own self-worth. Ellin describes visiting her grandmother for summer vacations as a child, a grandmother who, after weighing the two of them every afternoon, said, "Girls have to be thin and beautiful." She always linked the two adjectives together. Ellin reports that her grandmother worried that one day, "I'd blow up like an elephant."

When puberty hit, Ellin gained twenty pounds in less than a year. She hadn't seen her grandmother in almost as long when she came for a visit. Ellin recalls that she overheard her grandmother telling her mother that "I'd become tremendous." She remembers reaching for a second slice of bread at dinner. Her grandmother slapped her hand away and said, "You don't need another." She said, "How can you let yourself go like this? You have such a gorgeous face. Don't you want boys to like you?" Then came the warning: "You need to lose ten pounds or you can't come to Florida." However, as Ellin says, "I didn't lose the weight and I didn't get to go to Florida that Christmas." Ellin reports that she spent the next six summers in various fat camps trying to make Grandma happy. "When I was heavy, I wouldn't visit her. When I was thin she would lavish praise on me as if I were royalty. 'Hello, Skinny!' she'd beam. This both pleased and annoyed me. I desperately wanted her approval and yet I resented her for making weight an issue. I was only a kid and I wasn't that big."[21]

At first glance, the lives of these two teens are far removed. Dylan lives in poverty and is on his own much of the time. His mother is obese. His only positive outlets are fast food, cigarettes, and TV. School is a burden, even a nightmare. He is just a kid trying to get things right in a tough world, and it's not working. The teen Abby Ellin describes seems not to be impoverished. She can take vacation trips to Grandma's house and attend summer camps, even if they are for "fat kids." But a family member faults her about her weight, and she is seemingly forced to always view herself in terms of gaining or losing pounds.

What they have in common, as do many overweight and obese teens, is the search for a place to either hide from the assaults on their weight or find some trusted adults who understand their plight and have the skills to help them and maybe the Margos, Kyles, and Kates of the world. Sometimes those skills involve teaching teens like Abby how to confront a loving family member, like her grandmother, and say "enough is enough," backed up by the support of the trusted adult educator.

Here then are two pictures of what it is like for teens from different backgrounds to be obese or overweight. When the American Heart Association suggests that attacking the obesity problem means focusing "extra attention upon those of greatest risk," I suggest we are talking about the Dylans and the Abbys of the world who can be found each day in our large secondary schools. But what does "focusing extra attention" really mean for educators? Is there a "focusing extra attention" model for them to follow? And how do we motivate more schools to embrace an "extra attention" model so they can reach all the Dylans and the Abbys?

Here is a vignette that describes in very specific terms how educators can help Dylan—and in the process Margo, Kyle, and Kate—to redirect their lives. It's a vignette that is based on a comprehensive education and intervention model involving a team of caring and skilled school and community professionals as well as support staff and the school, students, and parents. This vignette is a composite of obese students I have counseled and of caring educators who were able to redesign their intervention system with the goal of not letting one student fall through the cracks, educators who acted on behalf of overweight and obese students, not just paying lip service to the slogan "no child left behind."

This vignette, then, is a story about how this intervention model is designed to help every teen in the school resolve his or her personal, health, and well-being problems, such as being overweight or obese. This intervention model is not built around a few savior teachers who operate on their own but on a team model that utilizes the helping resources of all members of the school community and in the process offers many open doors for help. It's a model that is proactive and ready and set to intervene at the first signs of a troubled teen. It is a model designed to serve every teen who meets trouble in his or her life, such as verbal assaults on weight. It is not a crisis model used to respond only to an immediate threat—potential suicide by a distraught teen, a sudden drug overdose by a straight-A student, or abuse of alcohol at a school dance. This "focusing extra attention" model is just that: intervening, educating, supporting, monitoring, and including and using the helping skills of recovering students.

The vignette also points out why being obese or overweight is a quiet problem in the schools. As I suggested earlier, the major survival goal for obese teens is to hide from peers, teachers, and administrators. Being invisible never really works for obese teens, but that's what many strive for. They understand from their own life experiences that when you stay out of sight, behind closed doors and in the dark, no one can verbally or physically abuse you. Your peers can't find you. It's a small victory in the battle to survive. Many obese teens know that finding a safe place in the schools, an arena of comfort, can be a daily challenge. Hanging out in the bathrooms behind a locked bathroom door can be such a safe arena: no mirrors in the johns to reflect your problem, just the sound of flushing toilets, the smell of a student grabbing a quick cigarette, and the coming and going of peers. Time passes slowly, but at least it's time when you're out of harm's way.

This vignette describes how schools can help the Dylans in our communities move out of hiding, out of the dark, and take their places as healthy and active students. But it is also a story about how skilled and committed individuals—educators, support staff, students, parents, and community advocates—can work as an effective intervention team, with each person expected to play a critical role in helping recovering obese and overweight students.

Dylan's story points out the need for educators to avoid limiting intervention to providing healthier foods in the cafeteria, teaching about healthy foods and diets, offering nutrition education for parents, and calling upon school staff to be models for healthy and active living. Surely healthy foods need to be made available to replace

17

the steady diets of burgers, hot dogs, and French fries that dominate the menus in many schools. And this effort needs to include teaching students about proper nutrition in every school venue—academic classrooms, physical education and health classes, group and individual counseling sessions led by school nurses and guidance counselors, and ongoing workshops made available by teams of health and physical education teachers, school nurses, and guidance counselors. And, of course, this effort needs to involve educating parents about proper nutrition and healthy diets.

However, I believe this intervention plan will fall short of its promise if educators ignore the need to provide individual and group support for overweight and obese students who have suffered verbal and physical abuse because of their weight. Overweight and obese students need an arena of comfort so they can begin to learn how to lose weight and be more physically active, and just as important, build their self-esteem, learn social skills so they can better interact with peers, family, and school staff, and be encouraged to have aspirations, hopes, and dreams. To recover, overweight and obese teens will require trusted adults in their corner who can provide a steady diet of emotional support and care—a teacher, coach, school monitor, nurse, assistant principal, or guidance counselor who is available and ready and set to guide recovering students like Dylan to sources of help. And they will benefit from the guidance of an older student, a big brother or sister, who has also fought to overcome a weight problem.

Simply put, while it is important to have cafeterias that offer healthy choices, educators who teach about the problems of being overweight or obese, parents who are savvy about nutrition, and staff who are models of healthy living, it is not enough. Schools also need to make sure that they have trusted adults in place to steer teens to sources of support, monitor and support their effort, and engage these students to help other students once they are healthier. It is not easy for teenagers to seek help on their own and form a plan to be healthier. Teens face many obstacles in turning a corner to make better lifestyle choices. The process of changing negative lifestyle habits, forming healthier peer groups, joining active school clubs and athletic teams, seeking positive adult role models, and dealing with the many setbacks that come when change is called for doesn't come easy without adult guidance and support. As can be seen in the case of Dylan, it takes many trusted adults to help turn a teen's life around.

Dylan's story begins in the office of Al Morris, an assistant principal at Moorhead High School. Al Morris, his staff, and Moorhead High are composites of real educators and schools I have observed. The work of Morris and his staff is an important reminder that there are educators and schools at the forefront of intervention to reduce obesity and related student health and well-being problems. There are intervention models such as the one at Moorhead High that educators can follow. Al is an energetic and caring administrator. A former English teacher and department chairperson, he's been at Moorhead for thirty years. He has seen the school grow from 900 students in grades nine through twelve to the current enrollment of 2,300. In his assistant principal role he oversees the discipline of 1,300 grade nine and ten students. Moorhead has a diverse student population that includes new immigrant students and students such as Dylan, on the move because of economic and family dislocation.

Al plays many roles in his position: disciplinarian, social worker, parent, teacher, preacher, coach, and confronter. He makes it his business to know each student, staff member, parent, and community advocate. He is quick to spot troubled students and direct them to staff members in the school who are skilled at intervening. He also relies on a cadre of student peer helpers who are trained in offering support to peers.

Al's plea to the faculty, students, and parents is, "I can't intervene to help every student. You have to help me by taking notice of kids headed for trouble, doing your best to connect with them, and guiding them so they get the help they need. You don't have to be a counselor to help. Just care about kids, talk to them, and be available and supportive. I'll provide the support you need and help you connect these kids with a counselor, psychologist, physician, whatever they need to stay out of harm's way."

Al's office is always crowded. He deals with many issues, most of them explosive: students who are fighting, tardy, cutting class, truant, abusing tobacco, alcohol, and drugs, bullying, having family problems, failing classes, and wanting to drop out, and new students who are not fitting in, like Dylan. Al is already getting reports on Dylan because of his cutting class, smoking, and being bullied by peers. The 1,300 ninth- and tenth-grade students at Moorhead carry many personal, health, and well-being issues into the school each day, and Al is the key player in helping them resolve these issues so they don't negatively impact on the students' academic performance.

As Al suggests, "Troubled students don't usually do well academically. Our job is to help relieve them of their troubles, whatever they may be, and get these kids back on track. At Moorhead we need to be vigilant and not turn our backs on one kid or look the other way when we see them headed for trouble. Ignoring a troubled student can be contagious. Once we ignore one troubled student, then it's easier to do the same for other students. That kind of behavior can kill the helping and caring spirit in our school. We need to avoid that trap at all costs. Otherwise, all we are here for is to teach our subject, pick up our paychecks, and go home. But effective teachers do more than just teach. Effective teachers know their students well—what their home life is like, their dreams and aspirations, the subjects and activities in which they do well, those subjects and activities in which they need support before failure sets in, and the personal and well-being problems they may be trying to solve. That's the teacher role that we have worked hard to create at Moorhead. It's a role that each of us has to work hard each day to hang on to, a role we are proud of, a role that makes Moorhead different. We are a school that values knowing and helping students and each other."

Dylan is in good hands. He has landed in a school setting in which staff, students, and parents are expected to take notice and, as the American Heart Association suggests, "focus extra attention." As in most cases, the process of focusing extra attention often begins with a classroom teacher, in this case Dylan's homeroom teacher, who mentions to Al that "Dylan is obese and always looks tired and acts tired. Plus he is starting to cut class, and some of the students say he is hanging out in the bathroom on the third floor. The kid is just taking up space. He clearly doesn't want to be here and doesn't want to fit in with his peers. And they know it and are beginning to turn on him. He stands out in the crowd as a kid who wants out of here. Now. We better move quickly or I have a feeling that we are going to lose him. My guess is that one day he is simply not going to show up. Maybe you could check on his background so we can begin to make a plan to help him. He sure is tough to get involved."

And so the intervention plan begins with a concerned teacher taking notice and focusing some extra attention on Dylan. The concerned teacher knows that in sharing her concern with Al, action will follow. Dylan's previous school record pretty much confirmed the teacher's assessment of Dylan. His parents are divorced, and his dad has no ongoing contact with Dylan. The family has moved many times, and Dylan has been in two different schools in the past three years. He missed over thirty days in his last school but still managed to pass every subject except physical education. His record indicates that he's had a number of referrals to counselors and school psychologists for being a "loner" and "isolated from his peers." The referral reports simply describe Dylan as "bright but lacking motivation and social skills." But much to Al's surprise, none of the data mentioned Dylan's weight as a possible source of his troubles in school. It was time for Al to meet with Dylan and assess the situation face to face.

Dylan was not surprised when he received the note in homeroom to come by the assistant principal's office after first period. It was a familiar story to him. New school and they want to know all about you and why you hate being here. Dylan thought, "I wish I had the balls to tell this guy that the kids are bugging me, I hate being here, and I am sick and tired of all the crap that comes my way in school. Not just this school but also every other school I've gone to. I just want to go home and never come back. Look, Mr. Al whatever-your-name-is, just leave me alone and stop trying to get to know me. Who knows how long I'm going to be in this school. Save your breath and energy for the other kids. I don't need you peeking into my life."

When Dylan showed up in Al's office, he didn't have to say a word. Al knew instantly the kid was having a tough time and every school day was probably a nightmare for him. He could see Dylan was very obese, maybe 280 or 300 pounds, and he looked very tired. And anxious. He was carrying around a lot of emotional and physical baggage for such a young kid. Al didn't waste any time getting to the problem. In addressing Dylan he said, "It looks like you're having a tough time fitting in, Dylan. Some of our teachers are concerned and I am getting reports you are cutting class and hanging out in the third-floor bathroom. I think we'll talk frankly about a plan to make things better for you at Moorhead. I know you've had your troubles in other schools you've attended, but here at Moorhead we want to help make you a healthy and successful student. Why did I say healthy? This isn't going to come as a surprise to you. You are clearly overweight and that's got to be causing you to feel terrible. Plus you look tired and anxious. Like coming to school and going through the day is one big hassle. Bottom line, to me, it looks like you can't continue on this path. I was an obese kid myself and believe me, I know how it feels to get the verbal and physical abuse that obese kids get. I hated school. But I was lucky. I had a counselor who guided me into healthy eating and activities where I lost weight and became a good student and athlete. My parents were divorced, like yours, and I was lucky enough to find a trusted adult like my counselor, Jack Morrison, who was like a father figure to me. I wouldn't be where I am today without his help. That's his picture on the wall, standing next to me with my high school diploma. So I know your story and I am going to help you. I don't want a 'no' from you. You know you're headed to some kind of health problems if things don't change. It's time to stop hiding out in the bathroom, cutting class, and missing school, and that time is right now. You are going to spend the next few hours with me, getting you the support you need to begin feeling healthier and boosting your self-esteem. Tell me if I'm wrong, but I can see your self-esteem is pretty low and your energy level is way down. You are running on empty, and unless we help you, you'll be on your way to dropping out. I think I am right on target. What do you think?"

Dylan was caught off guard by Al's aggressive invitation. In the other schools all the administrators and counselors did was talk about how he needed to shape up and be responsible. Dylan could still hear the words: "You are bright. Don't you want to be successful and go to college?" But this guy, Al, was, as he said, right on target. "He's been there, as a fat kid like me," Dylan thought. "Shit, I've got nobody in my life except Mom, and she has enough to do. I am tired, as Mr. Al said, and he is right, I feel like I'm running on empty. I am cutting class and locking myself in the bathroom. I am hitting bottom. Sitting there smelling the urine and stools just to avoid class and the hallways. Maybe I've found a way out."

Turning to Al, Dylan said, "OK. You are right on target about me. The truth is, I've tried to lose weight and I can't. And I've tried to fit in with the other kids, but I'm no good at it. I sort of lost my hopes and dreams. Like going to college and being a coach. All I seem to do is move from town to town and school to school. People see I'm unhappy, but they look the other way in disgust. I haven't belonged in a long, long time. Yeah, I'll go along with your plan. Thanks, Mr. Morris. My mom will be glad to hear about this. She's been very worried about my weight and school stuff. Could you give her a call sometime so she knows I'm getting some help? She'd really be relieved hearing from you. And maybe you could give her some advice about my brother Kyle and sister Kate, who are in junior high. They are having a tough time, too."

Al Morris is very skilled at interventions. He handles Dylan with care but also is very direct. He wastes no time in seeking Dylan out once a teacher raises a concern. He addresses Dylan's problems up front and essentially tells Dylan, "Look, kid, you've got some problems. But so do many other students here at Moorhead. Let us help you. You've got everything to gain and nothing to lose. You do want to feel better, don't you?" Al's invitation is compelling. In this role he is salesman, preacher, and a human being who has had weight issues himself and can relate to Dylan on a personal level. And he doesn't let Dylan off the hook once he makes a commitment. He grabs his coat and tells Dylan, "We are off to meet some special people in the school. I believe they are going to be a big help to you and maybe your mom. I am excusing you from third and fourth periods. You'll learn a lot in the next few hours. By the way, I haven't had breakfast. Let's begin our walk with some breakfast in the school cafeteria. I hear you go out to McDonald's for lunch. Maybe once you meet with Ms. Clifford, our nutritionist, and see what's available for breakfast and lunch, you'll think about eating in."

Dylan is beginning to get the extra attention he needs in small doses as Al Morris begins bringing him face to face with the trusted adults and students who will be his support group. Al knows the personal touch works with staff and students. No e-mails or memos about Dylan's "case." He knows that showing up in person with a needy student in hand sends the message that this student is a priority and needs attention right now. And showing up in person also sends the message to staff that Al Morris believes they are just the people to help this kid.

The first stop on Al Morris's intervention trek is the school cafeteria. The cafeteria at Moorhead has recently been reorganized. In a real sense it is trying to make a comeback and offer a healthy alternative to students who go off campus to eat lunch at the many fast-food chains that surround the campus. When Moorhead High was build in 1955, the enrollment was 900 students, and every student ate in the cafeteria. In 1967, with the enrollment soaring, an addition was put on the school so that it could house 2,500 students. Moorhead High now houses over 2,300 students and is nearing full capacity. During the late 1960s and early 1970s, Moorhead, like many large urban and suburban high schools, had student unrest. Student protesters called for the right to be allowed to go off campus during lunch and free periods. As a result, student abuse of tobacco, drugs, and alcohol increased, as did eating disorders spawned by daily diets of fast food. However, the new emphasis in the late 1990s and early 2000s on the need for schools to intervene to help students solve their personal, health, and well-being problems has begun to change the ways schools feed, teach, model, and, when necessary, intervene to promote healthy lifestyles for students and parents.

While understanding that it would be unrealistic and a losing battle to return to a closed campus, Al Morris and the school's new Wellness Team, made up of key teacher, student, parent, and community leaders, decided that the best approach to teaching students about healthier eating would be to redesign the school cafeteria so that it might offer an alternative to the fast-food chains. They wanted to send the message that Moorhead staff was serious about offering healthy alternatives to its students.

So when Al Morris and Dylan walked into the cafeteria, they found a setting with bright colors, festive pictures, and a computer lounge to do research while eating, a lounge for listening to CDs, and an attractive buffet menu offered throughout the day featuring natural juices, fruits, cereals, vegetables, grains, cheese, and low-fat milk products. Yes, there were pizza, fries, and burgers to satisfy the fast-food crowd, but they were made with healthy ingredients. The room that was once the staff dining room was now renamed the Got a Question Room. Staff were now expected to eat with students as a way to model healthy lifestyles. The room was staffed each lunch period by one of the school nurses, guidance counselors, or physical education and health teachers, who offered workshops, one-on-one counseling, and referrals when needed. Community health and mental health professionals also offered workshops and referrals on health issues. The "Get Yourself Healthy" bulletin board in the cafeteria cited special intervention programs in the school and community, with their phone numbers. These included the 48-Hour Program that students could enroll in to help them stop abusing tobacco and drugs as well as get support with other health issues such as overweight, obesity, anorexia, and bulimia, and also the 5-Hour-a-Day Program to help students reduce their tobacco smoking during the school day and learn to change unhealthy lifestyles. Next to the bulletin board was a bookcase containing handouts on health issues such as addictions, unsafe sex, sexual and physical abuse, family violence, and so forth.

Over breakfast Al suggested to Dylan that the cafeteria was a place where Dylan could learn important information about healthier eating habits, dieting, help with stopping smoking, and where to find help in the future. He suggested that Dylan sign up for a weekly tutorial class taught by the cafeteria nutrition specialist, who could also give him information about eligibility for the school breakfast and lunch program, since his mother might qualify. Kyle and Kate might also be eligible.

"Mission accomplished," thought Al. "Dylan knows where the cafeteria is, will get the information he needs on eligibility for the breakfast and lunch programs, and will be under the wing of Nancy Clifford, the nutritionist, and most important, he will meet other students with weight issues in the tutorial class."

The next stop for Al Morris and Dylan is a visit with ninth- and tenth-grade school nurse Barbara Grant and student assistance counselor Brad Langdon. Al has had his secretary call ahead to alert them that he would be dropping by with a student in need. Barbara has been at Moorhead for ten years, after a long stint as an emergency room nurse. She is a strong advocate for student health issues and for early intervention. Brad is a recent addition to the Moorhead counseling staff as a result of a reorganization that divided the staff into five major counseling roles: college guidance, testing, scheduling students for classes, career guidance, and personal, health, and wellness counseling. Brad is a recent Ph.D. graduate in school counseling and brought with him the latest approaches in one-on-one and group counseling and intervention. Some veteran members of the guidance program did not welcome the reorganization and, according to Al Morris, are still offering resistance to the new format. But the school administration, members of the Wellness Team, parent and community advocates, and students themselves were demanding reorganization to address the many different needs of students and parents. Brad has weathered the resistance and after two years on the job has won over most of the resisting counselors as well as students, staff, parents, and community advocates. Barbara and Brad's offices are located side by side with the intent that they would team together to offer a variety of intervention services to students.

In the meeting with Barbara and Brad, Al asked them to tell Dylan about some of the interventions they could provide to help him with his weight and self-esteem issues. Both Barbara and Brad offered to see Dylan separately in one-on-one sessions each week. Barbara suggested that they begin to monitor Dylan's weight, blood pressure, daily diet, and smoking habits if needed, and that they connect him and his mother to a community clinic where his cholesterol and blood sugar could be regularly checked. Barbara also mentioned that both she and Brad headed up the 48-Hour Program, offering support over the weekend for students trying to lead healthy lives, that is, to avoid tobacco, alcohol and drugs and eat healthy foods. Barbara told Dylan that once he absorbed all this new support, he might want to consider joining the 48-Hour Program. Brad suggested, as did Barbara, that once Dylan felt comfortable in the one-on-one counseling sessions and began to make his way at Moorhead, he might want to consider some other options, such as joining a support group to teach students about how to improve their peer relationships and perhaps joining the school peer counseling program that met after school. Brad indicated that the goal of the peer program was to train students in how to help peers who are headed for trouble, by teaching them how to listen, observe, intervene, and guide students to sources of help in the school and community.

Finally, both Barbara and Brad asked Dylan if they could set up an appointment with his mother in order to talk with her about the interventions for Dylan and how they might be of help to her and Kyle and Kate. Barbara said that she was in weekly contact with the school nurse at Kyle and Kate's school and maybe they could talk about some possible interventions for them when their mother came to the school. Barbara also added, "Dylan, we know your mom is very busy. Mr. Langdon and I will arrange our schedules to meet her needs. She comes first!" Then, turning to Al, Brad said, "You've probably already thought about this. Tony Jankowski and Marge Edgar have just introduced a whole new wellness curriculum in their physical education classes. I noticed in Dylan's record that he isn't doing well in his PE class. How about my changing his PE class and placing him with Tony and Marge?"

Al said, "Great idea, Brad. The gym is our next stop. I believe Tony and Marge are both teaching this period. Thanks so much for your intervention ideas and support for Dylan and his family. You two are a great combo. Keep up the good work."

Al was running out of time. He knew his office would be crowded with students, staff members, and parents wanting, sometimes demanding, resolutions to their problems. Resolutions in their favor most times. The past weekend there had been drinking at a homecoming dance, and he had had to suspend twenty students on Monday. Suspensions for drinking alcohol on school grounds as well as using drugs and alcohol required that students attend a mandatory ten-session workshop led by Brad Langdon. Some of the students who were suspended were straight-A students, on the honor roll, and star athletes. He would be dealing with this issue for weeks.

But Al knew he also had to be visible and out in the school and helping kids. He was grateful to Dylan for giving him this opportunity. Al had decided early on in his role as assistant principal not to be glued to his office and forced only to react to problems. He wanted to be a visible model for intervention, not a seldom-seen administrator who dished out only discipline, not hope. Al understood the pressure to handle both these roles. His secretary had called him four times about problems during his trek with Dylan. It was what it was, and it wasn't going to get easier.

Physical education teachers Tony Jankowski and Marge Edgar had persuaded their chairperson, Mark Donnelly, to allow them to embark on a model program to help improve students' health and well-being. They had won a grant to buy machines to monitor and record blood pressure, weight, physical activity, and so forth, creating an ongoing wellness profile for each student. The system would flag potential health problems for students who might require intervention. The grant also enabled the team to purchase a variety of exercise machines to help encourage regular exercise for students. In fact, when Al and Dylan walked into the gym class, Dylan said, "This looks like a health club." Tony and Marge, both members of Moorhead's Wellness Team, had long tired of physical education classes being labeled as "just throwing out the ball and letting the kids play." They believed that while exercise and developing a healthy lifestyle had become a priority in the community, the schools were lagging far behind in providing the same kind of intervention for students.

The need for such intervention was well known. Students who have healthy diets and exercise on a regular basis tend to be healthier and happier; have higher self-esteem; are less apt to be overweight or obese and less likely to abuse tobacco, alcohol, and drugs; and live longer and more productive lives. Tony and Marge worked closely with nutritionist Nancy Clifford, nurse Barbara Grant, counselor Brad Langdon, and health professionals from the community clinic and St. Charles Hospital. When a student like Dylan appeared on their radar screen with obvious health problems, they were ready to act quickly to provide both school and community intervention. Al suggested to Tony and Marge that Dylan would be moving into their class the next day. Al also mentioned some of the planned interventions suggested by Nancy Clifford, Barbara Grant, and Brad Langdon.

The plan for Dylan was in place. Al planned to speak with Martha Mayer, Dylan's homeroom teacher, about the plan before she left school. Recently the school had adopted an advisory system in which homeroom teachers were trained to serve as quasi-counselors for students, that is, to be a trusted adult who knows each student well, recognizing their aspirations, hopes, and dreams as well as areas in which they need intervention, such as academic and social skills; personal, health, and wellness issues; and family problems. The advisor's role was to serve as watchdog on the front lines of the school in order to identify students headed for trouble. Martha had surely done her homework in telling Al about Dylan. She needed to be congratulated for sharing her concern and given a spotlight at the next advisory training session. Finally, Al needed to contact school psychologist Harry Polk. Harry was chair of Moorhead's Child Study Team. The team was made up of the school nurses, counselors, special education teachers, classroom teachers, and administrators. The team met once a week to monitor the progress or lack of progress of students identified as needing intervention. Al needed to alert Harry about the planned intervention and make a presentation at the next Child Study Team meeting.

Before heading home that night, Al made a list of the interventions planned for Dylan, data he could use in his presentation to the Child Study Team. He also planned to send copies to Nancy, Barbara, Brad, Tony, Marge, Martha, and Harry. Here is his list of interventions:

- Al Morris will contact Dylan's mother about the intervention plan and Dylan's eligibility for free breakfast and lunch and alert her that she will be hearing from the school nurse and student assistance counselor.

- Dylan will be encouraged to eat breakfast and lunch on campus.
- Dylan will receive information on eligibility for free breakfast and lunch from Nancy Clifford.
- Dylan will attend Nancy Clifford's tutorial on healthy eating and diet.
- Nancy will try to connect Dylan with Moorhead's Farm-to-School Program, which uses local farm products in the cafeteria menu. The Farm-to-School Program employs needed students on weekends to help prepare food products shipped to the school.
- As part of the nutrition tutorial, Nancy will try to connect Dylan with peers who will be positive role models.
- Barbara Grant will meet with Dylan once a week to monitor his weight, blood pressure, and so forth; counsel his mother to help Dylan attend a community clinic where his cholesterol level, weight, and blood sugar will be monitored; and serve as an ongoing health resource counselor for Dylan.
- Barbara Grant will encourage Dylan to join the 48-Hour Program to help him maintain a healthy lifestyle on weekends.
- Brad Langdon will meet with Dylan each week to offer one-on-one counseling.
- Brad Langdon will encourage Dylan to join a support group designed to help improve social skills and also to become a peer counselor.
- Barbara and Brad will meet with Dylan's mother to apprise her of their intervention, provide information on community health and mental health support services, invite her to become involved in a parent support group led by Barbara and Brad, and offer to make outreach to Kyle and Kate's counselors in the junior high.
- Tony Jankowski and Marge Edgar will involve Dylan in a daily regimen of exercise and encourage him to participate in intramural or other athletic programs in the school and community.

- Martha Mayer will continue her ongoing support efforts with Dylan and provide feedback to his mother, the Child Study Team, and teachers on his progress.
- Harry Polk will make Dylan's case a priority with Child Study Team members.

Is this kind of intervention taking place in many of our large secondary schools? From my observations as an education reformer, I must say the answer is a resounding no. This is not a blaming statement but rather an assessment of where we are in our school intervention services. However, I believe this kind of intervention model to help overweight and obese teens and teens impacted by personal, health, and well-being issues described in the vignette is very doable. The data are in. As Bill Gates suggests, the model for the American high school is obsolete. High schools were designed fifty years ago to meet the needs of another age. Gates advises, "Until we design them to meet the needs of the 21st century, we will keep limiting, even ruining, the lives of millions of Americans each year." And as Gates suggests, "But these are our high schools that keep letting kids fall through the cracks, and we act as if it can't be helped. It can be helped. We designed these schools; we can redesign them. The basic building blocks of better high schools include making sure kids have a number of adults who know them, look out for them, and push them to achieve."

Dylan is a teen falling through the cracks. In his previous schools he's been a victim of an outdated process in which intervening to help troubled teens is the responsibility of an already overwhelmed small cadre of counselors. The intervention process in these schools moves at a snail's pace. Counselors are charged with the impossible mission of providing college counseling, testing students, scheduling students for class, and providing career guidance and outreach to parents. Intervention to help troubled students like Dylan is often offered only if there is a crisis such as a suicide attempt, a death of a student, a drug overdose, alcohol or drug abuse on campus, violent altercations between students or between students and staff, and so forth.

As Gates suggests, the Dylans in our schools slip through the cracks in this system. They are highly skilled at not being known, with a "leave me alone" sign posted on their faces and bodies. They represent a quiet problem. They are invisible, they hide, and they don't make waves. And they have a long history of saying no to offers of help. They don't want their troubles and stories known and their parents involved. They understand that in most schools, once they visit the assistant principal's or counselor's office, they are off the hook, able to get lost, be anonymous among their 2,300 peers. There is no Al Morris, Barbara Grant, Brad Langdon, or Martha Mayer to pursue, challenge, and confront them, to help them become aware that the troubles they are experiencing are not going away without help. They need the intervention of caring educators like Al Morris to convince them there is no escaping the gravity of their situation unless they, like Dylan, take an offer to help, an offer from a trusted adult who sends a message that says, "Come with me, let me help you, all will be well again." That offer doesn't come to many overweight and obese students in many of our secondary schools because there is a long line of troubled peers already formed outside the offices of a few counselors. Often the parents of these students are not participants in the school process. They may work two jobs and don't have time for PTA meetings; workshops on parenting, health, and nutrition issues; open houses; or meetings with teachers during the school day. In many schools these parents are labeled as not caring or as those who need the parenting workshops but never show up.

In the end, if Dylan doesn't get the intervention he needs, he is on the road to dropping out of school and becoming an adult who, as Gates suggests, could become one of the "one in four [who] turns to welfare or other kinds of government assistance." But more seriously, if Dylan doesn't get the intervention he needs, he is on the road to a lifetime of poor health and an early death, on the road to a diminished future with his days consumed by inactivity, illness, and worries about his welfare and Medicaid being wiped away. It's a bleak picture, a picture in which everyone is losing—Dylan, Margo, the caring and overwhelmed counselors trying to help but locked in an intervention system designed to meet the needs of another age, administrators and staff members who have grown tired of ineffective intervention efforts, troubled students who see no open doors of help and support, and parents like Margo who look to the schools for intervention for their children but find only closed doors.

Yes, as Gates says, "Everyone agrees this is tragic." But saying "this is tragic" is no longer good enough. We can no longer ignore the personal, health, and well-being problems of teens. As California superintendent Jack O'Connell points out, there is a clear link between health and well-being and academic success. We have to move beyond the outdated vision of a few counselors charged with helping to solve the health and well-being problems in schools with thousands of students. We need to redesign our intervention models with an emphasis upon developing an intervention team made up of many members of the school and community—like Nancy Clifford, Barbara Grant, Brad Langdon, Tony Jankowski, Marge Edgar, Martha Mayer, and Harry Polk. We need education leaders like Al Morris who are models for staff, students, and parents on how to intervene and help troubled teens, who respond to changing times by encouraging a redesign of the outdated cafeteria, hiring a nutritionist, implementing a teacher advisory program to help forge closer relationships among staff. We need leaders like physical education chairperson Mark Donnelly, who gave the green light and support for Tony Jankowski and Marge Edgar to redesign the physical education program to, as Bill Gates suggests, "meet the needs of the 21st century." I would add to Gates's statement that we must also meet the needs of parents like Margo and teachers like Tony Jankowski and Marge Edgar, giving them support to provide their children and students with the skills they need to lead healthy and active lives.

There are personal and career risks in taking the lead to redesign our intervention efforts to combat teen obesity and related problems. For example, Al Morris stepped out of the historical role of the assistant principal. He views himself as a facilitator and model for help, not simply limiting his role to reacting to the never-ending student problems found in our large high schools. Al gets out of his office and walks the talk with teaching staff, students, support staff, and parents. As he says, he knows his people. That means he can spot signs of trouble coming from staff, students, and parents. The bottom line for Al is that he understands that fewer troubled students will end up in his office if they receive early intervention. He understands that the level of safety, academic test scores, and staff, student, and parent morale will increase when the number of troubled students is reduced. He understands that obese students like Dylan quietly consume a great deal of staff time, such as checking on class cutting, calling parents, requiring him to go to summer school if he fails, resolving conflicts with bullying peers, and suspending him for smoking.

Al knows that a healthy and successful Dylan translates into more available time for him, Barbara, Brad, Martha, and other staff to help other teens headed toward the margins of school life. I believe Al is right on target with his analysis of time spent in redesigning our secondary schools. There is a lot of time being wasted in our schools by not finding efficient ways and models to help troubled teens like Dylan, hard-to-reach parents like Margo, caring teachers like Martha Mayer who are not given the skills they need to help troubled students, and cafeteria staff workers reduced to offering vending-machine food and drink with no hope or plan to compete with fast-food chains.

The risks for Al are very real. He spends time out of the office. He is feeling the political heat from veteran staff members because of his focus on being in the hallways rather than being in the office like the former assistant principal. These vocal veterans are sounding off in the faculty room and in the community about the school's Wellness Team taking away the staff lunch area and making it into a resource center for troubled kids. As one teacher was reported to say, "Twenty years ago we would have forced some of these kids to leave and join the Army when they screwed up. Now we coddle them. And who loses? Teachers like us who are thrown out of their own lunchroom." Some of the guidance counselors are angered over creating Brad Langdon's student assistance counseling position and providing advisory training for teachers. As one counselor said, "Al and the administration are turning over our jobs to this new kid with a Ph.D. and no experience and training teachers to advise kids. Pretty soon they won't need us." They have taken their concerns to the teachers' union, which is always on guard to save jobs. Many veteran teachers are uneasy with the effort to redesign the organization of the school by bringing in new roles and personnel such as Nancy Clifford and Brad Langdon.

Al's efforts do come at a cost. He is a target, something that often happens to leaders when change is necessary. But as leaders like Al understand, or need to understand, that while most staff members at Moorhead would agree with Bill Gates that it is tragic to let students like Dylan fall through the cracks, getting them on board to redesign the school organization they have known for many years is usually strongly resisted. Organizational changes to help students like Dylan are not always easy. Yes, Al is at risk, just as his troubled students are. He no longer enjoys the perks of his English department chair and teaching position, such as observing and helping teachers, teaching students, and leaving school unburdened. There are no easy days. He has moved on to a new level where the learning curve is much steeper and where good intentions for helping students often get waylaid by self-interest and political turf.

The remaining chapters deal with how we can proceed to put in place the various components that make up an effective early-warning intervention system that can quickly respond to overweight and obese teens and help them resolve related personal, health, and well-being problems. I argue that while schools cannot control all the factors that go into a teen's becoming overweight and obese, what schools can do is to identify these students; intervene; monitor their health indicators such as weight, blood pressure, and so forth; have the cafeteria provide alternatives to the fast-food chains found around most large schools; engage students in a rigorous regimen of daily exercise and physical activity; offer counseling and support for the students and their families; and involve these recovering teens in activities such as peer counseling where they have the opportunity to help others.

As the Centers for Disease Control and Prevention (CDC) states, although the primary mission of schools is education, neither students nor staff can be successful when health-related factors interfere with learning and teaching.[22] Increasingly, the educational attainment of every child, leaving no child behind, is one of our nation's highest priorities. Those with the responsibility of improving academic outcomes recognize that unless educational institutions address the health-related needs that compromise students' ability to learn, students cannot reach their potential as sound, productive citizens. By addressing health-related issues, schools not only foster students' academic achievement but also help establish healthy behaviors that can last a lifetime.

Young people spend more time in school than in any other social institution but the family. Researchers have identified protective factors that can reduce health risk. These include students' sense of "connectedness" to their schools and their access to community resources. The degree to which students feel positively connected to school is strongly related to whether they achieve academically. In the school setting, behaviors are developed and reinforced that will govern actions for a lifetime. The lessons students learn in school about high-risk behaviors can affect not only their present health and their success in school but also their health and productiveness as adults.[23] About 49.6 million students filled the schools in the United States in 2003.[24] Educators have a captive student audience and a unique opportunity to help them become and remain healthy citizens.

Here is a chapter-by-chapter plan of how I believe we should proceed to help educators take advantage of this opportunity and in the process demonstrate how adding critical components to the schools' intervention systems can spur the redesign of our high schools for the twenty-first century.

- Chapter 2 focuses on how high schools have been unwitting participants in helping teens become overweight and obese and how schools can redirect the process. The chapter examines how a series of education reforms have had unintended consequences in the ways students eat during lunch periods and their relationships with trusted teachers. The reforms have led to the creation of open-campus policies in many large schools, policies that encourage students to leave the school building during lunchtime and use free periods to eat at the increasing number of fast-food restaurants surrounding our large high schools. In chapter 2 I lay out a plan for educators on how they can reorganize their schools in order to compete with fast-food outlets and lure a portion of the exiting students back to a school environment that stresses healthy eating, healthy lifestyles, and positive contact with teachers who are models for healthy living.

- Chapter 3 focuses on what educators need to teach students, parents, and staff about the health risks that come with being overweight and obese. This is the first step in the effort to lure exiting students back to the school setting and reclaim the territory and turf now dominated by fast-food restaurants. This chapter stresses that the process of getting the attention of high school students concerning the health risks related to a steady diet of fast food—high blood pressure, high cholesterol, heart and cardiovascular disease, diabetes, and so forth—cannot be abstract. In my counseling of high school students, I have found that lectures, handouts, and school assemblies with speakers who use scare tactics such as "you'll be dead by age forty if you continue to eat burgers and fries each day" have little chance of success in challenging the unhealthy habits of students. Why? The vast majority of students give little attention to their own mortality. They feel that what they eat, drink, or smoke will have little long-term impact on their lives. "When I get to be twenty-five" or "when I get pregnant" are often students' answers when asked when they are going to change their unhealthy lifestyles. While the primary goal of this chapter is to provide educators with the data about the risks involved in being overweight and obese, I stress that the best ways to convey these risks are in the informal conversations students have with a number of trusted adults in the schools, such as Al Morris, Barbara Grant, Brad Langdon, Tony Jankowski, Marge Edgar, and Martha Mayer. These trusted adults are informed about health risks and can act when they observe unhealthy students like Dylan. As I stress in chapter 2, it is the personal contact, modeling, and support that matter in changing students' unhealthy lifestyles.

- Chapter 4 focuses on how educators like Al Morris can spearhead an effort to revitalize their school cafeterias in order to compete with fast-food restaurants. In this chapter I stress that educators can learn a great deal from the success of these restaurants. For example, they are clean, they provide courteous service, there are no long lines, and they provide a limited but attractive menu. There are pictures, posters, up-to-date and colorful tables and chairs, and music playing in the background. Fast-food restaurants have an ambience that promotes a casual, hanging-out atmosphere for students. In talking with students I have found that many don't even mention the food. What matters is hanging out, being with friends, and having time to "just be." I believe we can create the same atmosphere in our school cafeterias and still provide healthy food. Teens will eat healthy food if it is available in a cafeteria setting that has meaning for them, where their presence is valued, where they will be missed if they are absent, and where they can laugh and joust with peers and faculty. The image I am describing of a revitalized cafeteria has roots in the family dinner that were more common in our long-past agrarian society, a place where children and adults came together to rest, relax, share stories of the day, joke and laugh, talk about hopes and dreams, losses and failures, and in the process eat a good meal. It's an image that is a stranger to many teens in today's hurried world. Chapter 4 lays out a format of how educators can recapture those positive feelings that come with dining together as a "school family."

- Chapter 5 focuses on how educators can revitalize high school physical education programs in order to encourage every student to develop a daily regimen of vigorous physical activity. It shows how to develop interventions that regularly monitor students' weight, blood pressure, cholesterol, body strength, and so forth; teach students rigorous exercise skills; refer students to school and community health resources when needed; and educate and inform parents about their children's physical well-being. In the process I highlight the skills of professionals like Tony Jankowski and Marge Edgar, who do more than just throw the ball out and let the kids play.

• Chapter 6 focuses on how educators can establish a Circle of Wellness in their high schools. It shows how to bring together the many different, and often competing, intervention resources under one umbrella, where they can operate as a collaborative team. In my experience with high school organizations I have found that student intervention resources, such as counselors, nurses, social workers, school psychologists, and teacher advisors, often operate on their own. In a time of tight school budgets and staff reductions, they have learned to guard their turf and promote the notion that their helping specialty is unique and to be valued. Their mantra might well be, "We don't cooperate or collaborate. We survive." While this response might be understandable in our unsettled times, I believe it is counterproductive for students, parents, and staff. I believe what is needed is a team effort in which every member of the school's intervention team has a role to play, a team in which the Barbara Grants, Brad Langdons, and Martha Mayers all know their roles and together provide a Circle of Wellness and an open door for unhealthy students like Dylan and his mother. I predict that attempts to create a Circle of Wellness will be met with great resistance from members of the school's helping professions. No one likes to give up turf that is hard-earned. Administrators need to be prepared for such resistance and have the skills and energy required to overcome the resistance. The health of our students is more important than allowing and enabling a number of isolated professional citadels with out-of-date intervention systems to remain alive in our schools.

• Chapter 7 focuses on how my proposed Circle of Wellness needs to include training staff to model healthy behaviors. Many staff will resist this effort. Some will say, "First they tell me my job will be teaching academics, then they say I am supposed to be a personal and health advisor to students, and now I am supposed to be a healthy model for students? What's next? I am no Mother Teresa. And they don't pay me enough." I argue that the administrative, professional, and support staff are necessary if we are going to stem the tide of teen obesity and that their inclusion is necessary to complete the Circle of Wellness, a circle in which no student or staff member falls through the cracks into an unhealthy lifestyle. It is obvious that these staff members are ideally positioned to model healthy eating, drinking, and exercise patterns as well as model the monitoring of weight, blood pressure, cholesterol, and so forth. Many students have parents who model unhealthy behaviors such as overeating, smoking, and drinking. If we talk about teachers being trusted adult models for students and being known to them, that is going to require staff stepping up and buying into this new role. Isn't it better to have healthy and well staff than unhealthy and lethargic staff, some of whom are overweight, obese, or suffering from a variety of health problems brought on by an unhealthy lifestyle? I believe that in our efforts to make our schools safe and healthy environments for students, we have not only overlooked the potential modeling power of staff but have also allowed some staff members to drift into unhealthy lifestyles associated with overeating, poor diet, substance abuse, and so forth. Why should they be deprived of learning a rigorous daily exercise regimen from Tony Jankowski and Marge Edgar? The health monitoring and counseling from Barbara Grant? The personal counseling from Brad Langdon? As I suggest in this final chapter, these are important and doable issues for leaders like Al Morris to consider. Administrators need to sell their staff on this vital role and convince them that they too have much to gain personally as well as professionally from being fit. Clearly the effort to help our students be healthier can also have the same rewards for staff. Serious illnesses and early death do not have to be part of the script for some educators.

NOTES

1. American Heart Association, *A Nation at Risk: Obesity in the United States* (Dallas: American Heart Association, 2005), 1–20.

2. Palo Alto Medical Foundation, "Teen Obesity," http://www.pamf.org/teen/health/diseases/obesity.html (accessed 30 Aug. 2005).

3. Palo Alto Medical Foundation, "Teen Obesity."

4. United States Department of Agriculture (USDA) Center for Nutrition Policy and Promotion, *Profile of Overweight Children* (Washington, DC: USDA Center for Nutrition Policy and Promotion, 1999), 1–3.

5. Centers for Disease Control and Prevention Fact Sheet (2003), *Physical Inactivity and Unhealthy Eating* (Atlanta: Centers for Disease Control and Prevention, 2003), 1.

6. Centers for Disease Control and Prevention Fact Sheet (2003), *School Health Programs: Promoting Healthy Behaviors Among Youth* (Atlanta: Centers for Disease Control and Prevention, 2003), 1.

7. Robert D. Putnam, *Bowling Alone* (New York: Simon & Schuster, 2000), 277, 283–84, 298, 302.

8. Laurie Tarkan, "Benefits of the Dinner Table Ritual," *New York Times*, 3 May 2005, F9.

9. Tarkan, "Benefits of the Dinner Table Ritual," F9.

10. Tarkan, "Benefits of the Dinner Table Ritual," F9.

11. American Heart Association, *A Nation at Risk*, 1.

12. "Comprehensive Bill to Truly Leave No Child Behind" (unveiling of Dodd-Miller Act 2003), http://www.cdfactioncouncil.org/ALNCB_reintrduction_PR.htm (accessed 6 Mar. 2004).

13. California Department of Education News Release, "State Schools Chief O'Connell Announces Release of New Publication Linking Student Health to Academic Achievement," http://www.cde.ca.gov/nr/ne/yr05/yr05rel147.asp (accessed 4 Apr. 2005).

14. Bill & Melinda Gates Foundation, "National Education Summit on High Schools," http://www.gatesfoundation.org/MediaCenter/Speeches (accessed 5 Apr. 2005).

15. California Department of Education News Release, "State Schools Chief O'Connell Announces Release of New Publication."

16. Roberta G. Simmons and Dale A. Blyth, *Moving into Adolescence: The Impact of Puberty Changes and School Context* (New York: Aldine De Gruyter, 1987), xii, 304, 351–52.

17. National Association of Secondary School Principals (NASSP), *Executive Summary of Breaking Ranks II: Strategies for Leading High School Reform* (Reston, VA: NASSP, 2004), 1–6.

18. Palo Alto Medical Foundation, "Teen Obesity."

19. Palo Alto Medical Foundation, "Teen Obesity."

20. American Heart Association, *A Nation at Risk*, 6.

21. Abby Ellin, "The Measure of a Woman," *New York Times Magazine*, 19 June 2005, 70.

22. Centers for Disease Control and Prevention, *Stories From the Field: Lessons Learned About Building Coordinated School Health Programs* (Atlanta: Centers for Disease Control and Prevention, 2003), xxi.

23. Centers for Disease Control and Prevention, *Stories From the Field*, 1–3.

24. The Associated Press, "School Enrollment Hits All-Time High," *Newsday*, 2 June 2005, A35.

2

HOW SCHOOLS BECAME UNWITTING PARTNERS IN HELPING TEENS BECOME OVERWEIGHT AND OBESE

I would like readers to keep in mind three important themes as they move through this chapter. First is *Fountain Hills Times* editor Mark Scharnow's observation, "Mistakes were made many, many years ago that now make it more difficult to change the [food service] system at Fountain Hills High School." The high school opened in 1992 with a school cafeteria seating 208 students. In 1998 it was predicted that by 2000 there would be 800 high school students and another 600 middle school students that needed to be fed.[1] Scharnow is right. Mistakes were made by many school districts in projecting adequate eating space for students.

Second, Greeley (Colorado) Central High School superintendent Tony Pariso advises, "If we can provide good food, kids are going to stay on campus, no matter if it's closed, partially closed or open."[2] I believe Pariso's advice is right on target. In my counseling work with high school students, I have found them to be savvy about the quality and pricing of food. They choose to eat where the food is good and at a place where kids want to be. Unfortunately, many schools have ignored the sound advice of Tony Pariso and made mistakes that have played a part in teens' developing unhealthy eating habits, patterns that have increased the risk for some teens of becoming overweight or obese.

Third, the advice of Robert Honson, director of nutrition services for Portland Public Schools in Oregon, is, "We can't be the school operation for fast food restaurants. We need to create a program that students accept and that has the nutritional integrity that you would expect from an educational institution. We decided to offer things that are unique. You can't just give things to students; you have to educate them. We teach the teachers and the teachers teach the students."[3]

Using hindsight we can now see that many school districts ignored the advice of forward-looking educators like Tony Pariso and Robert Honson and fell into the trap of making mistakes that limited their capacity to feed each student good food in an attractive environment where kids want to be. Here is the story of how mistakes were made and how schools can once again attract a percentage of students, if not all of them, back to campuses that serve nutritious and healthy food in an attractive environment.

A century ago, many students attended community high schools that had relatively small enrollments. They ate lunch in cafeterias staffed by local adults and ate from a menu that often included produce from local farms. Teachers often ate with their students and were in a position to serve as trusted adult role models who could intervene to stop overweight and obese students from being bullied. The cafeteria was like the community commons where students from every walk of life came together to communicate, be seen, and be heard, a place where students and teachers had informal conversations about sports teams, how their parents were faring after the divorce, scholarships available at the state university, and how former graduates were doing. Of course these conversations included informal advice for students with academic, personal, health, and well-being problems. In these small high schools, students and teachers were able to get to know each other on a personal level. In the process, teachers could identify teens who were headed for trouble, such as those with weight gain, a bruise on the face, a pattern of being tardy to school, the recent death of a loved one, and so forth. These small high schools made it easy for students to come in contact with a trusted adult who knew them well, who knew their hopes, dreams, aspirations, health, social and academic strengths, and areas that needed improvement. Many of these informal helping conversations took place in the cafeteria. There were few open campuses, and fast-food chains didn't exist.

But all that began to change in the 1950s, when James B. Conant, former president of Harvard, recommended that small high schools be eliminated and that no high school should have a graduating class of fewer than one hundred students. The new schools—Conant called them "large comprehensive high schools"—would be able to offer students many more academic options than small schools were able to offer and hopefully act as a strong force to raise academic standards and compete with the emerging threat from Russia signaled by the October 1957 launching of Sputnik, the first space satellite. That meant reducing the number of high schools in the United States from 21,000 to 9,000.[4] The movement to large comprehensive high schools had many unintended consequences for both students and teachers, such as changing the ways in which students and teachers interacted and ate together.

As I suggested, when students attended small high schools, they were known by many adults in the schools. They were not anonymous. However, in many cases students were bused long distances to attend the new comprehensive high schools. In school they interacted with large numbers of students from different communities. It became easier for students to become unconnected and be at the margins of the school. Students' anonymity was heightened by the fact that they found themselves eating in large cafeterias with many students they did not know, served by little-known staff members and lacking the close contact they had formerly enjoyed with cafeteria workers and teachers in their smaller schools.

As these large comprehensive high schools grew in enrollment, many chose to open their campuses and allow, some might say encourage, their students to eat lunch at the growing number of fast-food chains surrounding the schools. One might see it as a marriage of convenience with unintended consequences. For schools it meant there would be less pressure to expand the school cafeteria. Or, taking a darker view, it was an opportunity to cut their cafeteria budget by feeding fewer students and therefore reducing cafeteria staff. And it was a financial bonanza for the fast-food chains. They became the primary source of daily lunch and breakfast for students, serving a menu that was a major contributor to the increase in their weight.

The move to open their campuses to students also emerged because the social, cultural, and political eruptions in the beginning of the 1960s acted to further isolate students from personal and trusted connections that had been the hallmark of small high schools. As education historian Diane Ravitch reports, the 1960s began with no hint of the troubles ahead for schools and society. Educators enjoyed a keen sense of success and pride in the new comprehensive high schools. But that feeling fell apart in many high schools in the 1960s. Many large high schools were confronted with violence, disciplinary problems, and litigation. In an effort to reduce conflicts, students were increasingly left to fend for themselves without adult guidance.[5]

The school cafeterias in many high schools, once the center of school life where students and teachers came together to communicate, be seen, and be heard, became places filled with vending machines full of unhealthy food and drink, manned by scaled-back staff, and whose revenues were used by the schools to defray the cost of other school programs, such as athletic teams, as budget woes increased. The fast-food chains became the center of school life. And the open-campus concept, with its conspicuous lack of trusted adults on the scene, proved to be fertile ground for students to develop unhealthy lifestyle habits such as overeating unhealthy foods, smoking tobacco, and using and abusing drugs and alcohol.

The upheavals in our high schools in the 1960s that led to the open-campus movement had a double whammy for students. They lost a portion of the needed contact with trusted adults in the school, and they became exposed to health hazards that could have long-term negative effects. As research by James Coleman suggests, instead of seeing themselves as adult role models whom students would turn to for advice when they encountered academic, personal, health, and well-being problems, teachers and other adults were retreating from their responsibility of monitoring young people, leaving them without adequate supervision and without moral benchmarks.[6] As Ravitch points out, in the 1960s and 1970s the rates of drug and alcohol use among teens soared.[7] So, I would add, did the weight of some students due to a steady diet of fast food.

By the 1980s, Coleman's prediction of an American society in which many children are increasingly left on their own without needed adult guidance and role modeling became the norm. The exodus from the city to the suburbs, he forecast, meant busy parents would work far from home. As the home ceased to be the center of social life and became "psychologically barren," he said, women would join their husbands in the workforce. Children would remain behind, given the latchkey to an empty house, abandoned to their own devices, and lacking responsible adult supervision. Children would learn how to behave from other children and from the television and movies. Under such circumstances they would absorb myriad random cues about how to conduct themselves.

The image for many teens in the 1980s was attending a large high school with a student population of over 2,000 and living in a home in which both parents worked or in a single-parent home. Their parents had little connection with the school, the family did not eat meals together, and the children were left on their own, without adult supervision, to eat, watch TV and movies, and, in the process, be less physically active.

As a result, fast foods became the dominant source of food both during the school day and at home in the evening and a major contributor to the number of teens being overweight and obese. The scene was set for overweight and obesity to increase dramatically for teens in the 1990s. Kids left on their own in school and at home became fair game—a captive audience, one might say—for the fast-food industry, left to fend for themselves and look to TV, fast-food commercials, movies, and peers for guidance. Arkansas governor Mike Huckabee offers a candid picture of the problem facing obese students when he recalls his own childhood experience. The son of a fireman who spent his spare time working as an auto mechanic, Governor Huckabee, as he tells it, grew up in stultifying financial circumstances and mainly on starch. "When you don't have much money, you're not going to be able to buy a movie or go to a major league ball game, but you can have a second helping of potatoes. One acceptable way for a good Christian kid to delve into a chemical addiction without being thought of as inappropriate or evil is to go to the pizza buffet. Pizza, well, that's OK." The governor was, by his own admission, a pudgy child who struggled with batter-covered food and a rising body mass index.[8]

Other factors have contributed to the rise in teens being overweight and obese besides reliance on a fast-food diet at school and at home. In the 1980s there developed a growing consensus that something had to be done to improve education standards. The 1983 *A Nation at Risk* report called for higher standards and an increased academic emphasis for students. The report warned that schools had not kept up with the changes in society and the economy and that the nation would suffer if education were not dramatically changed. The report, prepared by the National Commission on Excellence in Education, focused on a host of indicators, all of which revealed a profound crisis in public education, with problems in the high schools receiving the lion's share of attention. The commission urged states and local school districts to increase the academic requirements for students seeking a diploma. The *A Nation at Risk* report was followed by an effort by the federal and state governments to increase standards and student achievement by mandating testing of students at every level.[9]

There were also unintended consequences in this move to increase standards and student achievement that were to impact on students' health and well-being to this day. Adding more courses and requirements for graduation meant that students had less time to eat in school cafeterias and for these cafeterias to become healthy alternatives to fast-food chains. It also meant that students had less time to play and for physical activity. As *Boston Globe* staff writer Anand Vaishnav reports, in many schools across the state children had to gobble their lunches in twenty minutes or less.[10] Representative John A. Spillotis of Peabody, Massachusetts, said, "Our children's physical and emotional needs are coming second to MCAS

[Massachusetts's state achievement tests] scores in our state right now. If children aren't eating enough and don't get enough physical exercise, then they are not going to get back to class and pay attention. They're going to be lackadaisical and lethargic."[11]

Abbreviated lunch periods have been a growing concern for parents and nutritional groups. Many schools have either reduced lunch time or kept it at a minimum and have boosted class time to respond to pressure to succeed on state tests. Representative Spillotis's push to mandate thirty-minute lunch periods in schools was supported by parents such as Ann Mitsopoulos of Peabody, who said, "We're trying to tell the kids not to eat ninety miles an hour, to chew and digest their food. And then we put them in school, tell them to hurry and eat and get back to class." But requiring a thirty-minute lunch period would mean taking time from somewhere else, said Nadine Binkley, Peabody's superintendent of schools. The system either would have to extend the school hours or take time from academics. Binkley said, "When you have a limited amount of time in the school day, and with all the mandates you've got to cover, something's got to give."[12]

What appears to be happening is the choice by schools not to take time from academics but rather push for a longer school day.[13] *Boston Globe* writer Scott S. Greenberger reports that Boston, Springfield, Cambridge, and at least seventeen other Massachusetts school districts are moving forward with plans to extend the day in some of their schools, rejecting the traditional 180-day, six-hour schedule because educators believe there is not enough time to teach students what they need to know. The twenty districts are applying for grant money from the Massachusetts Department of Education to explore adding about two hours to the school day in some schools.[14] I believe there is no guarantee that this increase in the school day would result in more time for students to eat. In this day of growing political pressure to increase standards and test scores, time for academics often receives top priority. But the move to increase the school day does bring with it the opportunity to have, as Patricia A. Haddad, cochair of the Massachusetts legislature's Joint Education Committee, suggests, "a far-reaching philosophical discussion we really need to talk about. Children need sufficient time to eat and schools should address health as well as academic issues."[15]

As a result of the move to create large high schools with open campuses; an erosion in America's connectedness, community involvement, and family life values and patterns; and the growing need to increase academic standards, student achievement, and testing of students, particularly in our large high schools, the eating pattern that has emerged for many teenagers is easy access to fast foods at home and off campus during the school day, less time to eat lunch, and the transformation of high school cafeterias from serving every student into scaled-back operations serving hurried students and those eligible for free breakfast and lunch, and providing vending machines that serve unhealthy food and drink.

According to a 2005 news release from the Center for Science in the Public Interest (CSPI), a 2005 Government Accountability Office (GAO) report leaves little doubt about the proliferation of junk food in America's schools. Despite pockets of progress around the country, the GAO report shows that nearly nine out of ten schools offer junk food to kids out of vending machines, in school stores, and via "à la carte" lines right in the cafeteria. High schools are pretty saturated with junk foods. The September 7, 2005, CSPI news release states:

> That some high schools have come to depend on revenue from junk food is a national disgrace. Strong federal action is needed to protect a major federal investment in the school lunch program. It's startling how many legislators have put the "rights" of Coke, Pepsi and other junk food makers ahead of the things that parents value, their kids' education and health.[16]

High school cafeterias that once served as the schools' community commons and connected students from diverse backgrounds, cultures, and neighborhoods, as well as being a setting for informal, positive faculty and student communication, also have been given a low priority and scaled back to reduce school budgets. As any observer of teen life can testify, high school cafeterias are no longer *the* gathering place for students. In comparison, school cafeterias at middle and elementary schools have a strong constituency that favors the serving of healthy food in an attractive environment. Many of these schools have active and vocal PTA members, like parent Ann Mitsopoulos of Peabody, who demand up-to-date foods and services for their children. High schools, with diminishing PTA enrollment and clout, don't face the same political pressures to provide healthy foods and up-to-date cafeterias for their students. As James Coleman predicted, high schools have become settings in which students learn how to behave from peers and from television and movies. They are left on their own in the new community commons, the fast-food chain, to absorb a myriad of cues on how to conduct themselves, where to eat, what to eat, and with whom.

As education reformer Deborah Meier suggests, the implementation of the *A Nation at Risk* report and subsequent demands for higher academic standards and student achievement have resulted in an increase in students' tuning out and dropping out for those at the bottom of the schools' achievement and academic ladder.[17] In my observations of high school students, "tuning out" translates into cutting classes and hanging out at nearby fast-food chains, settings that have become havens away from school and home, settings that for many students are places where they can find a sense of belonging and a temporary high from salt-laden burgers and fries. Anyone who has been on a diet of fast food knows the stuff works to give them a sudden jolt of pleasure. Combining that pleasure with the high that comes from smoking a cigarette can make the school cafeteria's offerings seem pale in comparison. As Arkansas governor Mike Huckabee suggests, a steady diet of salt, sugar, and battered food can be addictive. Throw in student tobacco use and other substance abuse, and the seeds for lifelong health problems have been planted.

It is no wonder that fast foods have captured the eating habits of high school students. Unintended consequences from a series of school reforms have until now put the personal, health, and well-being issues of teens on the back burner. The academic reformers have led the charge and succeeded. I argue that in the wake of these successes to improve standards and achievement, many politicians, educators, and parents are beginning to demand that schools address, as Patricia A. Haddad suggests, health as well as academic issues and that we engage in a far-reaching philosophical discussion about these issues. In many states and local communities there is emerging a vocal group of parents, educators, and community advocates calling for the closing down of the high school open-campus policy. They are witnessing an increase in student deaths due to auto accidents during lunch breaks, violent physical altercations between students and between youth gangs, students using and abusing tobacco, alcohol, and drugs, students returning to school in an agitated state brought on by reactions to high sugar doses in soda and food served at fast-food chains, and an increase of overweight and obese students triggered by a daily regimen of fast food. Often altercations and fights are a result of students' being agitated by a combination of high dosages of sugar, substance abuse, and the absence of trusted adults such as teachers who could quickly intervene to reduce conflict with students they know on a personal basis.

As writer Theresa Vargas reports, some high schools in Long Island, New York, are revisiting their policies of letting students leave school for lunch after recent fatalities and attacks. Vargas describes a number of incidents that have led to the reexamination of open campus policies. On November 16, 2004, seventeen-year-old Olman Herrera was stabbed to death as he walked back to Hempstead High School. On October 7, 2002, a Commack High School student, Garry Abbot, a seventeen-year-old senior, died and his passenger was injured when their car was struck by another car with three students inside. Abbot was returning to school after a lunch break. On October 28, 2001, four Herricks High School students died in a fiery lunchtime crash. They were killed when their car hit a van while heading toward a fast-food restaurant. According to Vargas, superintendent Alan Grovesman of the Connetquot, Long Island, schools suggests, "We believe children are safer in schools. I think parents are very happy with the closed campus policy as it stands."[18]

But many districts across Long Island allow students to leave for lunch. Some permit it across all high school grades. As *Newsday* reporter John Hildebrand suggests, off-campus privileges have led to loitering, fights, and traffic deaths. Hildebrand reports that Jericho High School has temporarily barred its 260 seniors from leaving school during free periods for lunch and coffee breaks because of the September 9, 2005, death of seventeen-year-old student Matthew Ravner, who was killed in the school parking lot shortly after he returned from lunch and fell off the running board of a friend's sport-utility vehicle.[19]

The deaths of students due to auto accidents and altercations between teen gangs receive most of the headlines about the need for schools to shut down their open-campus policies. But what is not talked about by school administrators is the lack of an up-to-date cafeteria service to serve as an attractive alternative to fast-food restaurants. Many high school cafeterias are like aging steel mills. They have been allowed to rust and become hollow shells of their once-prominent part of the school organization. Their decay is part of the deteriorating physical structure in many of our large high schools.

Writer Russell Nichols reported in 2005 that in Beverly, Massachusetts, Beverly High School's accreditation was in jeopardy. The New England Association of Schools and Colleges contended that Beverly High School had neglected to maintain its worn physical plant. Neglect had occurred even though the school of roughly 1,300 students had been improving academically for the previous five years and more than 70% of its sophomores scored at the highest level on the MCAS test the previous spring, higher than the state average. School officials agreed the school needed a makeover. In Massachusetts, Lawrence High School, as well as Jeremiah E. Burke High School and O'Bryant High School of Math and Science, both part of the Boston Public Schools, lost accreditation in the 1990s for shabby facilities, high failure rates, high absenteeism, and high dropout rates. It's no wonder that many students who attend high schools with out-of-date and shabby facilities flee when they can to attractive, clean, responsive fast-food chains. Maybe the diet of the fast-food chains is problematic, but the place works to respond to hurried students' need for a quick food fix.[20]

I argue that the large comprehensive high schools envisioned by Conant and education reformers have over time failed to gather support for increasing school cafeteria budgets and staff and the development of healthy menus to attract and serve a changing school population. In many communities there has been an ongoing cry for schools to cut their budgets even though student enrollment is rising. Often the first areas to be cut are the school cafeteria and repairs to the physical plant. It's no wonder then that many high schools depend on an open-campus policy in order to make sure their students are fed. As Hildebrand reports, the two high schools in Levittown, Long Island, release over 500 seniors each day for lunch. District school superintendent Herman Sirois says, "If we had our choice, we'd rather keep them all inside. It's a lot safer."[21] However, while 500 students going out for lunch each day to fast-food restaurants may be dangerous and unhealthy, it means big bucks for the community's fast-food chains and takes pressure off the schools to beef up their food service systems.

Bob Nolke, director of student affairs at Hickman High School in Columbia, Missouri, clearly spells out the problem many high schools face in feeding students. Hickman High School has an open lunch. This means that the students are free to leave the campus during their lunch period. According to KOMY-TV, for Hickman it is partly out of necessity. "We have about 2100 students here. Our cafeteria seats about 200. There's no way we can feed 2100 students in two lunch shifts," says Nolke. Although open lunch helps the overcrowding problem, it has several disadvantages. For instance, Hickman students must cross some of the busiest streets in Columbia to get to the nearest fast-food places. Nolke says the advantages seem to outweigh the disadvantages. The school does not have to build another building, and the students can eat what they want. Hank Landry, a teacher at Hickman, adds, "If you look around here, the hallways aren't very wide, the place was built a long time ago. There aren't a lot of amenities here for students. It's almost like a rite of passage. You get to Hickman and you can go out for lunch." Landry addresses the growing academic pressure on students and the lack of time in the school day to unwind. "A lot of these kids have six or seven straight periods that are fifty minutes each. They have five minutes in between periods. It is hardly enough time to go to the bathroom. If they can get outside and get some fresh air and a change of atmosphere, theoretically they may come back ready to go another two or three hours."[22]

The situation at Hickman is not uncommon throughout America. As Bill Gates suggests, as quoted in chapter 1, many of the high schools were designed fifty years ago to meet the needs of another age. Many of these schools have neglected infrastructures, such as school cafeterias, that can't or have chosen not to compete with fast-food restaurants. The result? Soaring enrollments have resulted in students being encouraged to eat off campus because the school food service system is broken or simply limping along. While more and more parents are calling upon the schools to provide better nutrition and increased physical activity, schools like Hickman are boxed in by a system that can't deliver, can't respond. The push to increase academic standards has resulted in reduced time for physical activity and eating and added more stress to the lives of students. Although Nolke suggests that the students can "get what they want" by eating off campus, he points out, "Many, many students do not leave campus. If you go out and look in our halls, our cafeteria and students lounge are filled with students eating, as are various places around the building that have food carts where students can get sandwiches and things. They sit on the floor and all over the place and have lunch."[23]

It appears that many students at Hickman want to remain on campus but, as Nolke states, "There is a need to expand the current lunch facilities but lunch rooms are not the school's priority. I would almost bet that our cafeteria facilities and things like that would be last on the agenda of things that are going to get done."[24] While the staff at Hickman may believe the open lunch is a "time when students can get what they want," a "rite of passage," and an opportunity for a "change of atmosphere" where "they may come back ready to go another two or three hours," the reality for students appears to be either opting for fast foods off campus or eating in crowded and outdated facilities without a "lot of amenities." In a quiet way this "how it's done here at Hickman" approach translates into some Hickman students being forced off campus or left to find a spot in the school where they can eat and unwind, a rite of passage that is not very attractive or very healthy for students. For caring educators like Hank Landry and Bob Nolke, the conditions at schools like Hickman mean putting the best face on a cafeteria system that is not only out-of-date but that provides no glimmer of hope and change, a system in which everyone loses out on healthy eating options—the students, staff, and administrators. The winners? The fast-food restaurants.

Not all open-campus eating policies emerge from overcrowded conditions. There are other factors at play in school boards' enacting of such policies. While many high schools' communications to parents say they have a closed-campus policy, in fact many students do leave campus at lunchtime and on their free periods. In some schools junior and senior class members have the privilege of going off campus if they "act responsibly." This policy has been a tradition in many schools for a long period of time. Educators in these schools say that allowing their students to leave campus for lunch teaches responsibility and prepares them for the soon-to-come freedom of college life. This policy, once in place, is hard to change, as Moorhead's Al Morris understood when he began putting together a new vision for the Moorhead food service system.

In addition, many parents are willing to give their children permission to leave campus on free periods and lunchtime. The reality is that while the Center for Science in the Public Interest states that 73% of high schools have closed campuses, many schools with a closed-campus policy in fact allow students to go off campus.[25] The policy of the Board of Education in Wichita, Kansas, states, "Pupils in grades eleven and twelve can leave campus as part of their lunch privilege."[26] The Pulaski County School District in Little Rock, Arkansas, has a campus policy that states, "The Board believes that the educational interests of District students are best served within the traditional structure of a regular school day. Therefore, the schools are not authorized to operate open campuses." However, the policy adds, "Local school rules may permit students in grades 10–12 to leave campus for lunch if conditions of safety, reasonable proximity to eating establishments, and community support are met."[27] In Greeley, Colorado, more than half of the high school students in the Greeley-Evans School District can leave campus for lunch despite a policy designed to keep them in school. About 1,350 high school students out of 2,400 in the district have received signed permission slips from parents allowing them to leave campus, even though the school board decided to close campuses in October of 1999.[28]

As described by writer Steve McClain, there is often a great deal of pressure on school administrators to maintain an open-campus policy from parents, students, and alumni. McClain reports, "Every day at about 12:20 PM the lunch crowd descends on the Big Sandy Pharmacy's grill and other restaurants in downtown Paintsville, Kentucky. But don't look for the coat-and-tie courthouse crowd. The more casually dressed seventh-through-twelfth graders from Paintsville High will overshadow them." Paintsville and a few other districts in the state allow their students to leave campus for lunch, continuing a tradition that officials there say teaches responsibility. "I think open lunch is one thing that attracts people to our district," says Bruce Dungan, a Frankfort Independent board member. "I think people want their children to go where they will learn to be responsible for themselves. As an alum, I'd hate to lose that." Principals at Berea, Frankfort, and Paintsville High Schools say the freedom that comes with an open campus helps keep students in check.[29]

It appears that in some schools students have what I would call the worst of both worlds, that is, opportunities to obtain fast foods in both school and community. In a "frequently asked questions" brochure to parents at both Wheeling and Buffalo Grove High Schools in Illinois, parents are advised that both schools have open-campus policies that allow students to leave the building for lunch. However, students who remain in the school to eat lunch in the cafeteria "can order from the fast food restaurants that bring food to the school."[30]

While growing safety issues are emerging in many communities that have open-campus policies, strong student and parent reaction to closing campuses often wins out, as was the case at Wausau East and West High Schools in Wausau, Wisconsin, in 2004. According to reporter Keith Uhlig, the Wausau School Board proposed lunchtime open campus for juniors, seniors, and second-semester sophomores at both high schools. Uhlig says administrators considered ending open-campus privileges after renovations at Wausau West's cafeteria, which allowed both high schools to have the capacity to serve their students on campus. They cited safety, an increasing drug use problem, and truancy as reasons to keep students at school and recommended a more restrictive proposal that would have allowed juniors and seniors to leave for lunch. However, according to Uhlig, students lobbied hard to keep the liberal open campus, saying that the privilege taught them to make responsible choices.[31]

While safety issues for students who go off campus for lunch and free periods is a growing concern in many school districts, they are often met with resistance. Reporter Tessa Hill reports that the Mesa Public School District in Mesa, Arizona, is debating the district's open lunch policies after a lunchtime car accident that killed two Dobson High School students in December 2004. Hill reports that the idea of closing the lunchrooms in all six high schools in the district raised questions among board members regarding existing facilities and how campuses could accommodate a higher volume of students at lunchtime. Board clerk Elaine Miner said, "Safety is an issue, but we also have to think about how academics will be affected."[32]

In a real sense the unintended consequences of earlier education reforms for large comprehensive high schools and the movement to open campuses that followed the turbulence of the 1960s have come home to roost and placed our students, educators, and schools in a dilemma. While more and more groups are calling upon educators to intervene to halt the rise of overweight and obesity among students, the reality is that many large high schools like Levittown and Hickman simply can't feed all their students. Many large high schools have been prodded to provide an open campus because of high enrollments, budget cuts, and student demands. Schools have been engaged in a contract with the devil in order to survive and quell angry citizens and students. Maybe it has not been intentionally or knowingly, but there has evolved an unwritten contract with fast-food chains in order for large high schools to survive. The schools need these outlets and the fast-food chains need the steady flow of dollars, a marriage of convenience rather than a marriage made in heaven.

The bottom line is that many high schools have come to depend on fast-food chains to feed students. We've outsourced our once-strong capacity to feed all our students. As the School Nutrition Association reports, a study of school and fast-food restaurant locations in Chicago found that 78% of schools have at least one fast-food outlet within a half mile of the school building. Half the schools, both public and private, have fast-food outlets within a third of a mile. The report emphasizes that schools with open-campus policies potentially undermine attempts to create healthy school environments by providing access to fast food in restaurants and convenience stores outside the schools. The report found that fast-food restaurants were clustered within a short walking distance from schools and that the number of restaurants available near schools far exceeded the number in areas without schools. In most of Chicago's schools, students can walk to a fast-food outlet in a little over five minutes.[33]

It is no wonder then that many high schools now find themselves hard pressed to offer a positive response to critics who are demanding that schools play a stronger role in helping students become healthy adults by providing healthy foods and diets. Not only have high schools outsourced their food services to fast-food chains but in the process schools have helped to create a culture in which many high school students feel they have the right to go off campus for breakfast, lunch, and coffee breaks. After all, eating out has become part of our modern American way of life.

Who can blame angry Jericho High School students who have historically enjoyed one-hour off-campus lunch breaks but who are now being forced to spend their free time in the school cafeteria, which many never visited, or the library? They've been schooled to think that while it may be dangerous and unhealthy to eat off campus, it is their choice and responsibility, not the school district's. They are not buying into the pleas from administrators and parents such as Joyce Novick, mother of a twelfth-grader at Jericho High School, who said, "I hate the idea our seniors have been majoring in fast food, instead of what they are supposed to do." The reality for Jericho students has been going out to lunch, a perk that has been enjoyed by every senior class at Jericho for many years. Selling these seniors on the need to put away the car keys, burgers, and fries and return to the cafeteria table is probably a lost cause. However, Jericho administrators' plan to turn part of the cafeteria into a senior eating lounge may be a beginning step to convince future seniors that there are trade-offs students need to make to remain safe and healthy. It's a hard sell, a hard sell indeed.[34]

The fast-food chains have arrived at a winning formula for capturing the eating habits of many of our teen students. In envisioning changes in our food services, I believe it is wise to identify why fast-food restaurants work for hurried high school students and consider adapting some of their organizational strategies for our cafeterias. First and foremost, fast-food outlets are usually clean, and service is prompt and courteous. There is no waiting in long lines to get served. The fast-food setting seems to have a comfortable ambience, with up-to-date and clean chairs and tables, pictures and posters on the walls, music playing, and an easy-to-read, limited menu. It's not like the school cafeteria many students avoid, a setting with worn chairs and tables, no music allowed, and long lines that eat into the forty minutes for lunch. It's a no-brainer for students to opt to eat at a fast-food outlet that is only a five-minute walk or a one-minute car ride away. Our work as educators is to rewrite the script we have helped create and develop a competing food service model that not only works as well for hurried high school students but also provides the incentive for them to be happier and healthier.

Open-campus policies have emerged for five major reasons:

1. Some schools lack the facilities to feed every student as enrollments have soared.
2. Some schools have simply found it easier and, they think, more cost effective to have students eat off campus. It eliminates the need for lunchtime supervision, cafeteria renovations, cafete-

ria staff, cleaning and waste removal, and complaints from students and parents about the quality of food served.

3. Open campuses have become a rite of passage and a tradition in many schools. Efforts to close campuses, even in schools that have developed the capacity to feed every student, are often resisted by students, parents, and educators who are accustomed to open-campus life.

4. As Gerald Tirozzi, executive director of the National Association of Secondary School Principals, suggests, principals are especially hard pressed to balance the pressure for higher test scores and teaching youngsters healthy eating and exercise habits. Tirozzi says, "On one hand principals know the value of nutrition and fitness, but they're not encouraged or rewarded to be leaders in this area."[35] According to Colorado's Mesa Public School District board clerk Elaine Miner, having an open campus in which students eat lunch in the community allows solid joint time in the schools to offer tutoring and club activities. In Boston, Massachusetts, the school day at Noonan Business Academy, one of three high schools formed from the former Dorchester High School, was extended by seventy-five minutes twice a week for freshmen to work on study skills, reading comprehension, and homework because the school posted the highest dropout rate in fourteen years for Massachusetts high schools.[36]

5. Many schools have failed to offer an attractive meal and free-time alternative, such as creating a meal and free-time environment in the schools where students want to be.

School policies clearly have played a major role in the exodus of students into the community. The inability to upgrade facilities, avoidance of taking responsibility for where and what students eat, opting to place the schools' emphasis on academics and raising test scores, giving lower priority to the nutrition and fitness of students, and failing to create an attractive mealtime environment in the schools have all contributed to students' unhealthy eating patterns. And, of course, taxpayers' and community leaders' lack of financial support have been the driving force behind these policies. *Fountain Hills Times* editor Mike Scharnow was on target when he suggested that mistakes were made years ago that make it more difficult to change the system, mistakes such as the limited capacity of the cafeteria. Fountain Hills High School's cafeteria, which seats only 209 students, was opened in 1992. In 1998 it was predicted that by 2000 there would be approximately 800 students, along with another 600 middle school students.[37] It's time to address the impact of such "mistakes" on the health and well-being of students in every community.

I argue that there are two critical factors at work in our schools and communities that may present an opportunity to encourage a percentage of students who go off campus back into the school cafeteria, as in the plan of Moorhead High's administrator Al Morris and the school's Wellness Team for attracting students with a nutritious and healthy menu in a pleasant and comfortable environment. As Steve McClain reports, Frankfort superintendent Judith Lucarelli advocates a plan to give high school students more options: "We're talking about having a cafeteria not looking like an elementary school, maybe the look of a food court. And if students feel like they need to stay to talk to a teacher during lunch, they can stay here and eat lunch without rushing to get to lunch and back."[38] There are alternatives that may encourage a percentage of students to buy into a healthy option to fast-food restaurants and stay on campus.

A unanimous vote of the members of the Blue Ribbon Open/Closed Task Force, which studied the open-campus policy at Durango High School in Durango, Colorado, urged high school officials to explore more ways to entice students to stay on campus. The Durango School District superintendent says, "The unanimous vote of task force members represents an interest in giving students the freedom to choose to stay on campus for lunch if they want."[39]

I have found high school students to be very savvy. Offer them attractive food that is tasty, healthy, and served by happy personnel in a food court environment and they show up. Offer them frozen pizza that costs more than a nearby pizzeria, served by a demoralized staff, in a cafeteria with worn tables, torn chairs, and peeling paint and in which the only students who come are those on free lunch with no money to go elsewhere, and they won't. Reporter Brian Griesbach describes a presentation by the Fountain Hills High School student government in Fountain Hills, Arkansas, defending the school's open-campus policy. Some of the key reasons for keeping the open-campus policy in place, the students noted, were that the prices of food in the cafeteria were too high, the quality of food was inadequate, and, as a video taken by the students showed, the food bins weren't stocked, there were long serving lines, and tables were messy.[40]

As a recent Gallup poll shows, students complain that the meals in their high school lunchrooms are poor or only fair and that most teenagers say they skip at least four out of five cafeteria lunches a week. According to Gallup, only one in three students, or 34%, give high ratings to the taste of a school cafeteria, with just 2% saying it is excellent. The Gallup survey has implications for fast-food restaurants and convenience-store chains that surround our large high schools, which are locked in a battle for the $3.7 billion educational market. Schools can become players in this battle if they offer an alternative that students see is in their self-interest.[41]

The second issue working in favor of our schools' being able to compete for students staying on campus for mealtimes is the issue of safety. While safety concerns in allowing students off campus have often been given low priority, I believe there is a growing awareness that open-campus policies not only contribute to the development of unhealthy eating patterns and weight gain for students but also raise the possibility of vehicular deaths; gang violence; alcohol, drug, and tobacco use and abuse; and truancy. Parents are becoming more concerned about where their children are, as are school administrators. Paintsville principal David Bolen has some concerns. He says, "It really concerns me we're turning 350 kids loose for fifty-two minutes."[42] And Frankfort superintendent Lucarelli says she "worries about students who drive. We have had reports of kids racing to get back to school because they take seriously not being late. And there are days when the weather is not good in the middle of the day when they get in their cars for lunch."[43]

I believe Mesa Public School District board member Rich Crandall offers the best approach to ensuring that students are safe. In response to the Mesa district's debate about closing the six high school campuses in the district after the deaths of two Dobson High School students while off campus, Crandall suggested that school cafeteria improvements are essential for students to be happy with a closed-campus policy. He said, "Before we make any changes, I would beg you to make serious improvement to get an environment where kids want to be there."[44] I believe Crandall's solution, creating an environment "where kids want to be there," is right on target. It is the most attractive and doable option for secondary school educators as they face three critical issues:

1. The growing need to revitalize their aging infrastructures and cafeterias
2. How to offer a positive response to the growing public clamor to provide more nutritious foods and increase physical activity for students without overburdening taxpayers
3. How to provide an attractive meal and free-time alternative to liberal open-campus policies that can result in the death of teens due to accidents; drug, alcohol, and tobacco use and abuse; truancy; and weight gain due to a steady diet of fast foods and sugary drinks

I believe that simply closing down open campuses without an attractive lunchtime alternative will bring only resistance and protests from both students and parent groups. As Joe Ogilvie, head counselor at Patrick Henry High School in San Diego, says, "Even if the campus is closed there will be kids who leave anyway."[45] But allowing open-campus policies to continue without regard to safety issues and, as Crandall suggests, an effort to create an attractive meal and free-time environment in the school where students want to be, such as the cafeteria at Moorhead High, also presents a risk to the health and safety for students. I argue that the only doable approach is creating an environment where, as Frankfort superintendent Lucarelli suggests, there are attractive options, options that will enhance the health of students but not overburden taxpayers.[46]

Blanket political mandates to close school campuses need to be scrutinized and countered if they result in schools' being forced into mealtime options that create problems rather than solve them. Recommendations from a Center for Policy Studies, Education Research and Community Development research report that school campuses should be closed and lunch required on school premises to reduce crime and violence during school hours need to be thoroughly examined.[47] In my assessment, the Memphis Shelby Crime Commission report that cites these recommendations fails to take into account what "lunch required on school premises" means for schools.

Closed campuses may lower the rates of crime and violence by students in the community during school hours, but at what price to existing school resources such as the school lunch program? Policymakers, educators, and parents need to ask, "Are there nutrition, health, and physical activity benefits for students in closing the campus, or is it business as usual?" They need to ask, "Why are schools in the business of playing a role in lowering crime and violence by students and not involved in delivering healthy food, nutrition, and physical activity to students during school hours?" The reality for many large high schools is that they are simply not equipped to handle large numbers and bring every kid back into the school for lunch. It's a no-win situation for educators, students, and parents. It's not a real solution for beleaguered administrators who on one hand are being criticized by parents and health advocates for not providing more nutritious food and physical activity for students while at the same time are being burdened by outdated facilities, food service systems, and physical activity programs.

As Fountain Hills High School board vice president Jim Dickey suggests, "I know we have some limitations in our facilities that preclude feeding every kid at the high school. Having an open campus is one way of alleviating that problem."[48] I argue that beleaguered school board members and administrators need to explore the creation of model programs such as Moorhead High's, a model that can help build public support and a political base by demonstrating to parents and students that schools are capable of helping teens develop a healthy lifestyle. And once teens like Dylan begin to get intervention on how to develop a healthy lifestyle, what can follow is a reduction in the number of teen deaths due to automobile accidents; alcohol, drug, and tobacco use and abuse; gang warfare; truancy; and crime and violence in the community.

I believe it is time to begin rethinking how educators can begin a process to connect students to healthy alternatives. The issue of how best to combat the epidemic of teen obesity is not simply about open campus versus closed campus. It's about what students eat in both settings and which setting has the best opportunity to feed kids healthy foods. Simply put, if schools are going to make the effort to teach students about how to develop a healthy lifestyle, they have to develop a place, a laboratory, where they can practice what healthy eating and nutrition are all about. That's how healthy eating patterns are formed. It must be practice that offers new learning and positive reinforcement, and that results in increased self-esteem, increased self-worth, and loss of weight for overweight and obese students. Let's remember Greeley Central High School superintendent Tony Pariso's advice, "If we can provide good food, kids are going to stay on campus, no matter if it's closed, partially closed or open." His comment goes to the heart of the debate about the role of the schools in providing nutritious and healthy food for students.

I argue that we don't have to settle for the current food service models found in our large schools, such as Hickman High, models that focus on minimum health and food requirements. At Hickman it appears that the major mealtime goal of Bob Nolke and his staff is to make sure every student "gets fed," whether it's at a nearby fast-food restaurant or in the crowded cafeteria or hallways. Getting students fed is what it's all about. Not what they eat, the way it's served, the amenities offered in the cafeteria, or the morale of the cafeteria personnel. Nolke has to make sure his 2,100 students are fed in any way he can. Chances are that Nolke and his staff have little time to consider healthy food alternatives without community support for revitalizing the school cafeterias. Clearly many caring educators like

Nolke have been left in a no-win situation. I argue, and I would guess Bob Nolke would agree, that there needs to be more to school mealtimes than simply getting kids fed if we are going to stop the epidemic of teen obesity.

As Robert Honson, director of nutritional services for Portland Public Schools in Oregon, advises, "We can't be the school operator of fast food restaurants. We need to create a program that students accept and that has nutritional integrity that you would expect from an educational organization. We decided to offer things that are unique. You can't just give things to students; you have to educate them. We teach the teachers and the teachers teach the students."[49] The good news in the battle to stem teen obesity is that we know that good nutrition and rigorous physical activity offered in the schools do play an important role in helping teens stay fit and healthy even when their lifestyles at home are lacking in these areas.

Here is how I believe we should proceed so that educators like Nolke and students at schools like Hickman can have the same healthy meals that teens in districts such as Portland have each day. I believe a plan to help get students on board in the effort to eat healthier foods and develop healthy lifestyles is very doable. Here is my eight-step plan:

1. The plan begins with a clear message and commitment by school and community leaders and health advocates to announce a plan to entice a portion of the students who eat off campus to begin using the school cafeteria. They will encourage students and their parents to consider that becoming and remaining healthy does involve trade-offs and critical decisions, and first and foremost of these decisions is where and what they eat. This plan should acknowledge that while the school may not have the capacity to feed every student, educators, parents, and community health advocates have made the decision to embark on a concerted drive to compete with the fast-food restaurants and retake a portion of the dining territory they now dominate.

2. School and community leaders need to admit that reforms in the school's organization have led to an open-campus policy and

served to drive students off campus and into the waiting arms of fast-food outlets. The school policies until now have been part of the problem of unhealthy school diets for students.

3. The plan should announce that there will be an ongoing effort to educate students, staff, and parents about the health risks for overweight and obese students. This is an education process that will help concerned students, staff, and parents to be able to identify students like Dylan who have weight issues and get them the intervention they need.

4. The school cafeteria needs to be revitalized. That will mean an effort to provide a menu of healthy foods, served by courteous and welcoming staff, in a setting that is up-to-date and attractive, not shabby, worn, and tired looking from years of wear. The goal is for the cafeteria to become a favored student destination and be able to market a product that can go toe to toe with the fast-food outlets.

5. The plan calls for a revitalization of the school's physical education program. It will become a program whose primary goals will be to encourage every student to develop a daily rigorous exercise regimen and to provide interventions to monitor a number of health indicators such as weight, blood pressure, body strength, and so forth. The program will also have the goal of working closely with the school nurse and community health groups to provide referrals for students at risk of health problems such as obesity and will feature outreach to parents in order to inform and educate them about their children's health and well-being.

6. The plan will feature an effort to reorganize the various professional, parent, and student intervention resources in the school that currently operate separately into a team effort called the Circle of Wellness. The Circle of Wellness will encourage collaboration and provide many open doors for students afflicted with personal, health, and well-being problems, such as overweight and obesity.

7. The plan will feature a concerted effort to involve staff in the Circle of Wellness by providing opportunities for them to de-

velop a rigorous exercise program, a healthy diet, and a healthy lifestyle. This intervention for staff is a natural progression. If the school is going to ask staff to be healthy models for students, then we have to provide them with the training, skills, and support they need and the knowledge that students, parents, and citizens do indeed depend on the positive health and well-being model they offer to students.

8. Finally, the plan involves a strong public relations outreach to sell students, staff, parents, and citizens on the cafeteria's new menu and related services. In my experience as an education reformer, I have found that promoting a new program entails a great deal of selling of the product to the various constituencies involved. This selling approach means targeting students, staff, parents, and community leaders in order to gain their support and provide concrete ways for them to get involved in the process. This may entail creating a school food service advisory board in which each constituency has a place at the table to offer its input. This selling process is not unlike a political campaign. For example, students, staff, parents, and citizens involved need information to understand the proposed changes, see that their own self-interests can be served by the change, and be called upon to be vocal and active supporters of the change.

Leaders, like administrator Al Morris and nutritionist Nancy Clifford, who want to revitalize their school food services need to keep in mind that convincing students that they are better served and healthier by opting to eat in the school cafeteria requires more than a timely idea, physical and menu changes in the cafeteria, and an assault on the dangers of fast foods. Winning the hearts and minds of students requires one-on-one and group contact with students—or focus groups, to use a political and media term—by key student, staff, parent, and community leaders. I believe this winning-over process needs to avoid angry and vocal confrontations with the fast-food restaurants. The school's effort to regain the dining territory of students needs to be a quiet sell based on the potential value of eating at the school cafeteria, not the dangers of fast-food diets. I argue, why make fast-food restaurants the enemy and in the process raise the possibility that students will come to their defense? After all, fast-food restaurants are what students have come to know and value. The reality is that the fast-food restaurants are successful at what they do, and although critics can rightfully say they offer unhealthy foods, the system works for them. They are simply doing what comes "naturally," serving food and making money.

In this selling campaign the onus is on the schools to offer an attractive alternative rather than bashing the fast-food outlets and inviting a student defense. What works is creating a positive alternative students can buy into. All the preaching in the world about the dangers of fast foods will go for naught unless teens have an alternative that offers the same ambience. The enemy in establishing better teen eating habits is not the fast-food restaurants but rather the inability of the schools to be creative enough to sell students on their product and services. To succeed in stemming the rising tide of students being overweight and obese, schools have to learn how to operate in the competitive world of food service, that is, to adopt a marketing approach that can convince students that the school can offer a better, healthier product than fast-food restaurants. I believe school leaders can learn a great deal from the political process in promoting this selling campaign. In politics a winning election often depends on the candidate's offering positive themes—selling the voters on the value of the candidate, what she or he brings to the office, and what is to be offered and using a platform that avoids focusing on negative themes and bashing of the opponent.

This selling campaign also requires a plan to target local resources for financial and political support, for example, alumni, local employers, colleges and universities, and community financial, medical, mental health, and media institutions. These might be resources that can donate furniture, kitchen equipment, staff uniforms, video and audio equipment, pictures and posters, cleaning supplies, health and food consultants, health and diet books and handouts, printing of menus and diets, and publicity in newspapers, TV, and radio. These donors can also help to fund the creation of a Health Honor Roll in cooperation with the school's wellness team. This honor roll would provide monthly awards for students and staff who have achieved success in such health indicators as weight loss, stopping or reducing tobacco use, lowering blood pressure and cholesterol, avoiding fast foods, and so forth. The awards would take the form of a written certificate proclaiming the health achievement and signed by school personnel and a monogrammed T-shirt supplied by a local vendor with the label "#1 Health Achiever." The names of students and staff honored with the awards would be announced in school and by the community newspaper, TV station, and radio station and be given a prominent place on the cafeteria's Health Honor Roll bulletin board. Dylan and Margo would be thrilled to have such an award to brighten their lives, something positive to hang on the refrigerator door and tell family and friends about.

Letting the school community know about the health successes of students and staff is an important part of the selling campaign. Students and staff need to know that some students, such as Dylan, are turning their lives around and that the school's efforts are paying off. In many high schools the health successes of students get little notice. What gets noticed and talked about are the problems and failures, the bad news. Success stories are limited to academic performance, test scores, class rank, college placement, achievement in athletics and the arts, attendance, and so forth. In most schools there are no report cards, honor rolls, and awards for students who achieve better health. In my own experience in attempting to reform school counseling, health, and physical education programs, I have found that if students and staff are acknowledged and affirmed for improving their health, they are often willing to come forward to tell their story, the story of how they went about the process and the positive impact these health changes have had on their personal lives and, for teachers, their professional lives. This opening-up process provides students and teachers with the opportunity to come out of the closet and become sources of hope, information, education, and role models for their peers. As part of this education process, their stories can be written and talked about in the school and local newspapers and on TV and radio stations.

In the end, if the school's selling campaign is to be successful, there needs to be a way for students and staff who are recovering their health to stand up and be known. We must put a real face on the statistic that among children and teens ages six to nineteen, 15%, almost 9 million children, are overweight.[50] The real face might be described in the Moorhead High School student newspaper: "In our school students like Dylan have worked hard to regain and maintain their normal weight thanks to intervention by staff such as Al Morris, Barbara Grant, Brad Langdon, Tony Jankowski, Marge Edgar, and Martha Mayer. Here is Dylan's story. . . ."

NOTES

1. Mike Scharnow, "Close the Campus During Lunch Hour," *Fountain Hills Times*, 21 Apr. 1999, http://www.fhtimes.com/times/1999archives/4-21-99/mike.htm (accessed 24 Oct. 2005).

2. Katherine Kennedy, "Closed Campus Poses Hurdles," *Greeley Tribune*, 12 Nov. 1998, http://www.greeleytrib.com/apps/pbes.dll/article?AID=/19981112?ONTHERIGHTROAD (accessed 23 Oct. 2005).

3. Carolyn Walkup, "National School Lunch Program Offers an Education in Nutrition," *Nation's Restaurant News*, 3 Sept. 1990, http://www.findarticles.com/p/articles/mi_m3190/is_n35_v24ai_8859786/print (accessed 23 Oct. 2005).

4. James B. Conant, *The American High School Today* (New York: McGraw Hill, 1959), 44, 78, 81, 93–94, 96.

5. Diane Ravitch, *Left Back: A Century of Failed School Reform* (New York: Simon and Schuster, 2000), 171–73.

6. James S. Coleman, *Adolescents and the Schools* (New York: Basic Books, 1965), 6–7.

7. Ravitch, *Left Back*, 239, 241.

8. Gina Bellafante, "The Governor Who Put His State on a Diet," *New York Times*, 10 Aug. 2005, F2.

9. National Commission on Excellence in Education, *A Nation at Risk* (Washington, DC: U.S. Department of Education, 1983), 18–26.

10. Anand Vaishnav, "School Lunches Are No Picnic," boston.com, 6 Aug. 2005, http://www.boston.com/news/local/articles/2005/08/06/school_lunches_are_no_picnic?mod. (accessed 6 Aug. 2005).

11. Vaishnav, "School Lunches Are No Picnic."

12. Vaishnav, "School Lunches Are No Picnic."

13. Vaishnav, "School Lunches Are No Picnic."

14. Scott C. Greenberger, "Districts pushing for longer school day," boston.com, 3 Oct. 2005, http://www.boston.com/news/education/K_12/articles/2005/10/03/districts_pushing-for-longer . . . (accessed 3 Oct. 2005).

15. Greenberger, "Districts pushing for longer school day."

16. Center for Science in the Public Interest, CSPI Newsroom, "Government Accountability Office (GAO) Report Shows Junk Food in 9 out of 10 Schools," 7 Sept. 2005, http://www.cspinet.org/new/200509071.html (accessed 17 Sept. 2005).

17. Deborah Meier, *In Schools We Trust* (Boston: Beacon Press, 2002), 1–25.

18. Theresa Vargas, "Schools' Open Question," *Newsday*, 13 May 2005, A39.

19. John Hildebrand, "An Open or Shut Case," *Newsday*, 2 Oct. 2005, A16.

20. Russell Nichols, "Beverly High School's Accreditation in Jeopardy," boston.com, 12 Oct. 2005, http://www.boston.com/news/local/articles/2005/10/12/beverly_high_schools_accreditation (accessed 12 Oct. 2005).

21. Hildebrand, "An Open or Shut Case," A16.

22. KOMU-TV, "Local Lunch Crunch," 22 Apr. 1997, http://www.missouri.edu/~kozlenk/lunch/lunch2.html (accessed 23 Oct. 2005).

23. KOMU-TV, "Local Lunch Crunch."

24. KOMU-TV, "Local Lunch Crunch."

25. Joy Johanson, "Nutrition Integrity in Schools," Center for Science in the Public Interest, 2004, http://www.cspinet.org/nutritionpolicy/fedschoolfood.pdf (accessed 4 Apr. 2005).

26. Wichita Public Schools, Board of Education Policies, July 1994, "Middle and High School Lunch Period Activities," http://www.usd259.com/policies/1358.html (accessed 23 Oct. 2005).

27. Pulaski County Special School District, Little Rock, Arkansas, "Open Campus," Board of Education Policies adopted 2 Aug. 2000.

28. Nate Haas, "Throngs of Students Leave for Lunch as Honor System Begins," *Greeley Tribune*, 19 Oct. 1999, http://www.greeleytrib.com/apps/pbcs .dll/article?AID=/19991019/ONTHERIGHTROAD (accessed 23 Oct. 2005).

29. Steve McClain, "Off-Campus Lunches on Menu for Some Schools," Kentucky School Boards Association, Jan. 2004, http://www.ksba.org/ KSA1004%20cafeteria.htm (accessed 21 Oct. 2005).

30. Community Consolidated School District 21, *Open Campus Policies at Wheeling and Buffalo Grove High Schools*, "Frequently Asked Questions," 2000, http://www.d21.k12.il.us/paths/faq_student.html (accessed 23 Oct. 2005).

31. Keith Uhlig, "Open Campus Stays," *Wausau Daily Herald*, 9 Mar. 2004, http://www.wausaudailyherald.com/wdhlocal/27999819863033 .shtml (accessed 23 Oct. 2005).

32. Tessa Hill, "Mesa Public School District (MPS) Debates Closed Lunches," newszap.com, 2 Feb. 2005, http://www.newszap.com/articles/ 2005/02/05az/east_valley/mesa03.txt (accessed 23 Oct. 2005).

33. School Nutrition Association, "Study Finds Fast Food Restaurants Located Near Schools," 12 Sept. 2005, http://www.schoolnutrition.org/ PrinterFriendly.aspx?id=1422 (accessed 13 Sept. 2005).

34. Hildebrand, "An Open or Shut Case," A16.

35. Rhea R. Borja, "Healthy Schools Summit Weighs in on Obesity," *Education Week*, 16 Oct. 2002, http://www.edweek.org/ew/articles/2002/10/ 16/07healthy.h22.html?print=1 (accessed 25 May 2005).

36. Maria Sacchetti and Tracy Jan, "High School Dropout Rate Reaches Highest in 14 Years," boston.com, 2 Oct. 2005, http://www.boston.com/ news/local/articles/2005/10/22/high_school_dropout_rate_reaches (accessed 22 Oct. 2005).

37. Scharnow, "Close the Campus During Lunch Hour."

38. McClain, "Off-Campus Lunches on Menu."

39. Dominic Weilminster, "Durango High School (DHS) Supports Open Campus," *Durango Herald*, 11 Mar. 2005, http://www.durangoherald.com/ news/05.news050311_1.htm (accessed 2 Jan. 2005).

40. Brian Griesbach, "Students Tell Board: Keep Open Campus," *Fountain Hills Times*, 30 Sept. 1998, http://www.fhtimes.com/times/1998 archives/9-30-98/open.html (accessed 24 Oct. 2005).

41. Rich Telberg, "School Feeders Turn Off Teens, Recent Gallup Survey Shows: Students Call Cafeteria Food 'Poor' or 'Fair,'" *Nation's Restaurant*

News, 14 July 1986, http://www.findarticles.com/p/articles/mi_m3190/ is_v20/ai_4353805/print (accessed 23 Oct. 2005).

42. McClain, "Off-Campus Lunches on Menu."

43. McClain, "Off-Campus Lunches on Menu."

44. Hill, "Mesa Public School District."

45. Sharon Jones, "Should Kids Stay on Campus for Lunch?" *San Diego Union-Tribune,* 8 Oct. 1995, http://debate.uvm.edu/eesample/090.html (accessed 24 Oct. 2005).

46. McClain, "Off-Campus Lunches on Menu."

47. Memphis Shelby Crime Commission, "Closed Campuses as a Strategy for Reducing Truancy," research report prepared at the request of Dr. Carol Johnson, Superintendent, Memphis City Schools, http://www.memphiscrime .org/research/studies/closed-campuses.html (accessed 23 Oct. 2005).

48. Griesbach, "Students Tell Board: Keep Open Campus."

49. Walkup, "National School Lunch Program."

50. Palo Alto Medical Foundation, "Teen Obesity," http://www.pamf .org/teen/health/diseases/obesity.html (accessed 30 Aug. 2005).

3

WHAT EDUCATORS
NEED TO KNOW
ABOUT THE RISKS FOR
OVERWEIGHT AND
OBESE TEENS

Over the last decades many high school educators have been trained to respond to a variety of student personal, health, and well-being problems that negatively impact on academic success: alcohol, drug, and tobacco abuse; eating disorders such as anorexia and bulimia; physical, sexual, and emotional abuse; suicidal thoughts; bullying; and family problems. Now, due to the nationwide focus on teen obesity, they are being asked to become knowledgeable about the risks involved for teens who are overweight or obese and how they can intervene and guide these teens to credible sources of help in the school and community, not turn a blind eye to these students, and to make intervention a priority.

As the American Heart Association recommends, we need to take action. The Associated Press reports that in 2005 more high school students in Indiana were overweight than two years before. From 2003 to 2005 the percentage of high school students considered overweight increased from 11.5% to 15%. The percentage of students who ate five or more servings of fruits and vegetables in the past seven days dropped from 20.3% to 15.5%. Milk consumption dropped nearly 5%. The survey showed that about 34%

of students did not achieve Centers for Disease Control and Prevention (CDC) recommendations for physical activity over a seven-day period, and 10.5% did not participate in such activity at all. However, their use of alcohol, tobacco, and marijuana declined slightly.[1]

The 2005 Youth Risk Behavior Survey released by the Indiana Department of Health was taken by 1,528 students in grades nine through twelve in fifty-three randomly selected Indiana high schools in the spring of 2005. It sought input in six categories: nutrition and weight, physical activity, tobacco use, drug and alcohol use, violence and injury, and sexual behavior.[2] As the Indiana study suggests, I believe educators are beginning to see some success in helping many high school students resolve their personal, health, and well-being problems. As in the example of Moorhead High School, some schools have pioneered successful intervention models. The next frontier is readying educators to confront the epidemic of teen obesity. That requires providing educators with background information about the risks for teens of being overweight and obese, information that will hopefully propel them to intervene, not look the other way, when they observe a teen on the road to obesity. The focus of this chapter is to provide educators with an overview of the information they need to know so they will be ready and set to intervene.

BEING OVERWEIGHT AND OBESE INCREASES MEDICAL COSTS

Overweight or obese Americans spend about $700 more per year on medical costs than trim individuals, according to a study by RTI International and the CDC. The study suggests that an obese person will likely spend 36% more on doctor visits and 77% more on medications annually. Every taxpayer shares the cost. That's approximately $175 per person. Being overweight or obese adds as much as $93 billion a year to U.S. medical costs.[3]

MANY OVERWEIGHT AND OBESE AMERICANS WANT TO LOSE WEIGHT AND ADOPT A HEALTHY LIFESTYLE

⎸According to *Time* magazine and ABC News, the weight problems of individuals have become a national crisis. Fully two thirds of U.S. adults are officially overweight, and about half have graduated to full-blown obesity.⎸The rates for African Americans and Latinos are even higher. From 1996 to 2001, two million teenagers and young adults joined the ranks of the clinically obese. People are clearly worried. A *Time*/ABC News poll released in June 2004 shows that 58% of Americans would like to lose weight, nearly twice the percentage who felt that way in 1951. But only 27% say they are trying to slim down, and two thirds of those are not following any specific plan. According to the *Time*/ABC News report, excessive poundage takes a terrible toll on the human body, significantly increasing the risks of heart disease, high blood pressure, stroke, diabetes, gall bladder disease, osteoarthritis, many forms of cancer, and psychological disorders including depression, eating disorders, distorted body image, and low self-esteem. The total medical tab for illnesses related to obesity is $117 billion a year and climbing. Poor diet and physical inactivity could soon overtake tobacco as the leading cause of preventable deaths in the United States.

Yet the report offers plenty of reasons for hope. Campaigns against smoking and drinking have raised the national consciousness about these public health issues dramatically. There is no reason to think that an antiobesity campaign could not do as well, as long as everyone involved acknowledges that the problem is real and that solving it will be difficult. Nature has stacked the deck against weight loss. Trimming twenty-five pounds from your figure may not be that difficult, but try shedding one hundred pounds and your body is going to scream.[4]

MANY OVERWEIGHT AND OBESE TEENS USE FOOD AS A SUBSTITUTE FOR SELF-ESTEEM

The *Time*/ABC News report suggests that although anorexia and obesity look nothing alike in clinical terms, there are similarities.

People with both disorders tend to organize their days around eating and allow food to loom large in their lives. Food for them is much more than a source of nourishment; it can become a substitute for self-esteem and a vehicle for exercising, or losing, control over the body. People with overeating problems are often successfully treated using diet and exercise and sometimes medications that curb appetite more successfully.[5]

SCHOOLS NEED TO DO MORE THAN SIMPLY LEAVE OVERWEIGHT AND OBESE TEENS TO TRIM POUNDS; THE PERSONAL RESPONSIBILITY APPROACH WITHOUT INFORMATION AND SUPPORT OFTEN FAILS

The *Time*/ABC News report suggests that for decades the country has seen obesity as a personal problem to be solved by overweight individuals waging a lonely war to trim pounds. The report concludes that the personal responsibility approach to weight loss has been a big, fat flop. What is needed is a change in our community and school landscapes, such as physical education classes, bike paths, accessible parks, and so forth. Dr. David Ludwig, a Harvard pediatrician, suggests that schools have become nutritional disaster areas. Students are a captive audience; promoting their physical well-being should be a part of the school's educational mission. Ludwig states that if we want to stop obesity, we have to stop building the infrastructure for obesity. We must eliminate junk food, fast food, and soft drinks in the schools. Ludwig's research shows that for every additional daily serving of a soft drink, a child's risk of becoming obese rises 60%. Ludwig suggests we need to reengineer opportunities for activity into our environment. We have many more schools than parks around the country. The challenge is finding ways to keep them open after hours as community centers.[6]

TEENS ARE BEING HOOKED ON JUNK AND FAST FOODS THROUGH A CONSTANT BARRAGE OF TV ADVERTISEMENTS

On December 8, 2003, ABC News broadcast a TV special, "How to Get Fat Without Really Trying," hosted by Peter Jennings, ABC's top news anchor. The show revealed some startling information on obesity. For example, the average American child sees 10,000 food advertisements a year on television; children spend more of their own money on food than anything else, more than on CDs or movies or clothes or toys; and in 2002 there were more than 2,800 new candies, desserts, ice creams, and snacks on the market but only 230 new fruit or vegetable products.[7]

A 2004 report by the Kaiser Family Foundation, "The Role of Media in Childhood Obesity," indicates that children who spend the most time with media are more likely to be overweight. However, contrary to common assumptions, more research reviewed for the report did not find that children's media use displaces vigorous physical activities. The research suggests that there may be other factors related to media use that are contributing to weight gain, such as children's exposure to billions of dollars worth of food advertising and marketing in the media. The report cites studies that show that the typical child sees about 40,000 ads a year on television and that the majority of ads targeted to kids are for candy, soda, and fast foods. The report also cites research indicating that exposure to food advertising affects children's food choices and requests for products in the supermarket. Other key findings of the report suggest that interventions that reduce children's media time and education campaigns to promote healthy eating and exercise result in weight loss for children and teens.[8]

LITTLE THINGS ADD UP FOR TEENS WHO WANT TO LOSE WEIGHT

Researcher Dr. Jennifer Zebrack advises that physical activity is vital to weight loss and a healthier body. She advocates choosing an activity you enjoy and can fit into your daily life. The little things add up, she says. "Take a walk around the block, reduce sedentary activities like TV, video games and computer use." She recommends that your goal for physical activity should be at least thirty to forty-five minutes per day, five to seven days per week. Dr. Zebrack also recommends that people eat their heaviest meal in the morning or at lunch, drink a glass of water before eating, eat more slowly, eat smaller portions, limit the number of meals eaten out (especially fast food), keep healthy snacks easily at hand, and get social support from friends, relatives, and mentors. Eating breakfast every morning may help teens maintain a healthy weight and do better in school. Recent research supports the importance of teens' eating breakfast. Researchers reviewed forty-seven nutritional studies and concluded that children and adolescents who ate breakfast had better mental functioning and better school attendance records than those who did not. And breakfast eaters, even though they consumed more calories, were less likely to be overweight.[9]

SCHOOLS HAVE BECOME UNWITTING PARTNERS IN HELPING TEENS BECOME OVERWEIGHT AND OBESE, BUT TIMES ARE CHANGING

According to author Gary Ruskin, years ago public schools were places where good nutrition was taught. In the 1920s, as part of the home economics movement, millions of school children were taught proper nutrition and which foods contained the nutrients they needed to grow. However, the curriculum of junk food nutrition began in earnest in 1989, with the launch of Channel One, an in-school marketing program. Chris Wittle, Channel One founder, had the ingenious idea of harnessing the schools to show daily TV broadcasts that included two minutes of ads. Since then, Channel One has been adopted by 12,000 schools. About 8 million children watch the ads for junk food, fast food, and soft drinks. Ruskin states that schools have become a paradise for junk food marketers. Vending machines stocked with candy and soft drinks are rife; nearly nineteen out of twenty schools have vending machines that sell soft drinks, and more than 70% of high schools sell chocolate candy in vending machines. Hundreds of school districts have signed marketing contracts in which the districts promise exclusive access to soft drinks, such as Coca-Cola or Pepsi, in return for financial incentives.[10]

The Center for Science in the Public Interest (CSPI) supports many of Ruskin's findings, indicating that 98% of senior high schools have vending machines, school stores, or snack bars that sell soft drinks, sports drinks, imitation fruit juices, chips, candy, cookies, and snack cakes. However, according to CSPI, there is strong support for improving school foods. A national poll by the Robert Wood Johnson Foundation found that 90% of teachers and parents support the conversion of school vending machine contents to healthy beverages and foods. Similarly, a 2005 *Wall Street Journal*/Harris Interactive Health-Care poll found that 83% of all adults think that "public schools should do more to limit children's access to unhealthy foods like snack foods, sugary soft drinks and fast foods."[11]

TEENS WHO DRINK TWO OR MORE SWEET DRINKS PER DAY ARE TWICE AS LIKELY TO BE OVERWEIGHT

According to the American Diabetes Association, teens have been eating more fast food since the 1970s. The association reports that teens who eat fast food take in more calories, more total fat, and more saturated fat. They eat very little fruit or milk and consume fewer important nutrients.[12] They also drink a lot of regular soft drinks with sugar.[13] They have higher body mass indexes (BMI) than people who don't eat fast foods. Overweight teens eat more fast-food calories than lean teens.[14] The association's data suggest that there is a strong correlation between being overweight and drinking one or two sweet drinks a day. Children who drink two or more sweet drinks per day are twice as likely to become overweight.[15] Based on information from the 2003 California Health

Interview Survey, researchers at the University of California at Los Angeles concluded that soft drinks play a major part in the daily diet of teens. The older teens get, the more soft drinks they consume. Seventeen-year-olds drink 40% more soda than twelve-year-olds. Boys drink 25% more soda that girls. Disparities also exist among racial groups and income levels. African Americans drink nearly twice as much soda and other sugary beverages as white or Asian youths. Latino teens drink 50% more soda than whites.[16]

The UCLA researchers suggest that soda and fast-food consumption goes up as household income decreases. Such foods are usually quick and cheap, making them especially appealing to families on a tight budget with both parents working long hours.[17] As the ABC News *Nightline* program of June 2, 2004, "Nightline: Critical Condition—Obesity Crisis," reports, "If you live in a low income neighborhood of Detroit, your family food budget is $25 a week, the nearest full-service grocery store is at least a bus ride away and on the way you pass twenty fast food restaurants, chances are you would have a serious weight problem."[18] As the UCLA research suggests, schools may be the one best source available to offer teens healthy foods and begin to guide them on a path toward reducing or eliminating junk and fast foods and beverages.[19]

INCREASES IN FAMILY MOBILITY AND IMMIGRATION HAVE HAD A NEGATIVE IMPACT ON FAMILY LIFE AND NUTRITION

The increases in family mobility and immigration have been contributing factors in many teens' becoming overweight and obese. According to author E. D. Hirsch Jr., mobility is high in our society. Hirsch states that about one fifth of all Americans relocate each year. In a typical community the average rate at which students transfer in and out of schools is nearly one third.[20] The rate of immigration is also soaring. Researcher James A. Banks reports that American classrooms are experiencing the largest influx of immigrant students since the beginning of the twentieth century. About a million immigrants are making the United States their home each year. More than 6 million legal immigrants settled in the United States between 1991 and 1996.[21] But simply stating that mobility is high doesn't capture the picture of families on the move. Joann Bellemore, found of the Big Beautiful Women Network, which organizes social events for obese men and women in Las Vegas, describes her childhood and teen years of being the only fat person in her family, the eldest daughter of a career Navy man and a strict Japanese mother who felt that an unwieldy body represented a lack of self-control. Like other military children, Ms. Bellemore spent her childhood bouncing around from city to city and from school to school. When she graduated from high school, she was five feet eight inches tall and weighed 235 pounds.[22]

As in Dylan's case, moving from community to community and from school to school can further disrupt an already fragmented family life. For parents there is the continuing cycle of finding work, finding a place to live, registering the children in new schools, arranging transportation to and from work, and so forth. The decisions and mini-crises never cease. There is no time for family dinners that focus on sharing the good and bad news of the day. Everyone is on the run. The TV and fast foods dominate their lives, providing a deadly cushion and escape from hectic lives. Immigration to a new country and community can also quickly disrupt healthy eating and lifestyles. As the *Time*/ABC News report suggests, among immigrants coming to the United States, the obesity problem has become a full-blown crisis.[23] Even the most stubborn of new arrivals may find that their food practices are impossible to maintain in a new environment, where familiar ingredients are not available, old-world holidays are not observed, and the Mediterranean tradition of a heavy lunch must yield to the less-healthy prospect of postponing the big meal until the end of the day. Newcomers share many of the problems that highly mobile Americans face, such as finding work, a place to live, and so forth, but many also face the reality of giving up food practices that provided a healthy lifestyle in their former country.

CHAPTER 3

TEENAGERS WHO ARE SERIOUSLY OVERWEIGHT TAKE A DIM VIEW OF THEIR EMOTIONAL, SOCIAL, AND PHYSICAL HEALTH

Education Week reports on research described in the April 9, 2003, issue of the *Journal of the American Medical Association* that suggests there is a growing awareness that the most widespread consequences of childhood obesity may be psychosocial. The research study involved 106 children between the ages of five and eighteen who had been referred to an academic hospital for evaluation of obesity. The study notes the similarities in the emotional, social, and psychological states of young cancer patients and obese children. Both categories of youngsters have trouble keeping up with their peers at school and participating in common activities such as sports. Moreover, they may suffer teasing and ostracism by classmates.[24] The American Diabetes Association also cites several studies that have shown that overweight and obese children and teenagers have a lower quality of life.[25] Surprisingly, teens who are overweight and obese are not immune to teasing and bullying by peers with the same afflictions.

Danielle Rothman, now seventeen, spent three summers at a camp for overweight and obese teens. Thousands of young people like Danielle spend their summers at weight-loss camps sarcastically labeled "fat camps." As Danielle reports, these camps can be hostile places: "Everyone at camp was overweight yet people were still made fun of because of their weight. The more overweight kids are still made fun of. I was one of the thinner kids and people would say, 'Why are you here?' It made me feel good but after a while I wanted to hit them."[26] As education writer Lindsey Tanner reports, even more disturbing is research that suggests that kids who are labeled "too fat" or "too thin" are more than twice as likely as normal-weight teens to attempt or think about suicide. The research study was based on a nationally representative 2001 survey of 13,601 students in ninth through twelfth grades. About 19% said they had considered suicide in the previous year, and about 9% said they had attempted it. The researchers said that because nearly half of the students *perceived* themselves as too fat or too thin, the results suggest that a sizable proportion may be at increased risk for suicide.[27]

As researcher William H. Dietz concludes, there are many psychological consequences to obesity. Children in kindergarten have already learned to associate obesity with a variety of less-desirable traits, and they rank obese children as those they would least like to have as friends. College acceptance rates for obese adolescent girls are lower than those for nonoverweight girls. Adult women who were obese as adolescents or young adults earn less, marry less frequently, complete fewer years of school, and have a higher rate of poverty than their nonobese peers.[28] Binge eating is also a problem for obese teens. Marsha D. Marcus's research on obesity suggests that between 20% and 30% of individuals seeking treatment for obesity regularly take in an objectively large amount of food with an associated loss of control over eating.[29]

THE RATE OF DIABETES IS SOARING FOR CHILDREN, TEENS, AND ADULTS

According to reporter Raja Mishra, obesity in the young has hiked type 2 diabetes cases. Type 2 diabetes, once called "adult-onset" and most common in those over forty, now accounts for almost half of new diabetes cases in U.S. teens. Almost all children with type 2 diabetes are overweight or obese.[30] Writer Jane E. Brody suggests, "I can't understand why we still don't have a national initiative to control what is emerging as the most serious and costly health problem in America, excess weight. Are our schools, our parents, our national leaders blind to what is happening, a health crisis that looms even larger than our smoking habits?" Brody states that the prevalence of diabetes nearly doubled in the American adult population, to 8.7% in 2002 from 4.9% in 1990. Furthermore, an estimated one third of Americans with type 2 diabetes don't even know they have it because the disease is hard to spot until it causes a medical crisis. An estimated 18.2 million Americans now have diabetes, but adults are not the only victims. More and more children are developing this health-robbing disease. Counting children and adults together, some 41 million Americans have a higher-than-normal blood sugar level that typically precedes the development of full-blown diabetes.[31]

Brody reports that a fifteen-year study published in January 2005 analyzed the eating habits of 3,031 young adults and found that weight gain and the development of prediabetes were directly related to unhealthy fast foods. The study suggests that consuming fast food two or more times a week resulted, on average, in an extra weight gain of ten pounds and doubled the risk of prediabetes over the fifteen-year period. Brody cites research by Dr. Francine R. Kaufman, the director of the diabetes clinic at Children's Hospital in Los Angeles and a past president of the American Diabetes Association, who states that in her first fifteen years as a pediatric endocrinologist, 1978 to 1993, "I never saw a young patient with Type-2 diabetes. But then everything changed. Teenagers now come into my clinic weighing two hundred, three hundred, even nearly four hundred pounds with blood sugar levels that are off the charts. But we cannot simply blame this problem on gluttony and laziness and assume that the sole solution is in individual change."[32]

According to Dr. Kaufman, other important factors in what she calls the "diabetes epidemic" are the failure of schools to set good examples by providing only healthy fare and the inability of many children nowadays to walk or bike safely to school or to play outside after school. Unless we change our eating and exercise habits and pay greater attention to the disease, more than one third of whites, two fifths of blacks, and one half of Hispanics in this country will have diabetes.[33] As Lisa Sanders, MD, describes, one of the lessons she learned in treating an adult male patient who weighed 350 pounds is, "There is a tendency in medicine to focus on the data about the patient, the vital signs, the monitors, the lab reports, rather than on the patient himself. We look after patients without looking at them. Thus the patient's obesity, an essential reason why he came to ICU, was almost forgotten as we tried to get him released. Doctors are really only beginning to appreciate the way obesity can affect a patient."[34] I would add that educators, too, are only just beginning to appreciate the way obesity can affect students.

SOME SCHOOLS ARE BEGINNING PROGRAMS
TO SCREEN STUDENTS FOR BEING OVERWEIGHT
AND OBESE

Writer Martha Raffaele reports that beginning in September 2005 the Pennsylvania State Health Department is requiring school nurses to complete students' body mass index, or height-to-weight ratio, during annual growth screening for children in kindergarten through fourth grade. Parents will get letters about the results that will encourage them to share the information with family doctors. The measurement will be required for students up to eighth grade in 2006 and for ninth through twelfth grade students in the 2007–2008 school year. About 36% of Pennsylvania's children are overweight or at risk of becoming overweight. Beth Trapani, spokeswoman for Pennsylvania Advocates for Nutrition and Activity, said, "Remedies to being overweight and obese are not complicated. We're talking about simple, easy changes that can make a big difference, such as low fat milk, eating more fruits and vegetables." According to Raffaele, A Chance to Heal, a Rydal, Pennsylvania–based advocacy group that supports the screening, argues that schools should be prepared to help children address weight problems by educating them about proper nutrition and providing adequate exercise time.[35]

Writer Roni Rabin echoes Beth Trapani's message that remedies for being overweight and obese are not complicated. Rabin describes the latest United States Department of Agriculture food pyramid for children, which calls for a daily diet of grains, vegetables, fruits, milk, oil, meat, and bean products.[36] In addition to Pennsylvania, other states have embarked on screening students for being overweight and obese. A research study in Arkansas that analyzed the body mass index (BMI) data of more than 345,000 students at all grade levels in 93% of the state's schools during the 2003–2004 school year found that 38% of students are overweight or at risk of being overweight. According to Dr. Joseph W. Thompson, the director of the Arkansas Center for Health Improvement, "No area of the state has been spared from the epidemic of childhood obesity. This study clearly indicates that children of every age, gender, economic status and ethnic group across the state are vulnerable."[37]

As a result, Arkansas enacted legislation, Act 1220, that requires an annual BMI screening assessment for all students in public schools, starting with prekindergarten. As in Pennsylvania, letters with individual results and suggestions to consult with a family physician were mailed to parents in the summer of 2004. The legislation also requires schools to disclose the details of food and beverage contracts and to remove vending machines from elementary schools. However, in both Pennsylvania and Arkansas, some parent and professional groups are offering strong resistance to the screening, suggesting that labeling or rating children as overweight can serve to humiliate heavier children, hurt self-esteem, and potentially increase eating disorders. These groups are also questioning the accuracy of the BMI. For example, they say the BMI can inaccurately cite athletic students as overweight because they have more muscle weight.[38]

Nutrition columnist Sally Squires suggests that the BMI often overestimates risk and cites research that the BMI was intended to screen populations, not individuals. She argues that the BMI should be used as a starting point, not gospel.[39] University of Virginia professor Glenn Gaessner, author of *Big Fat Lies*, points out, "While extreme obesity can be dangerous, the health threat of being overweight or obese has been exaggerated. I do think some scientists and the media have overestimated the risks."[40] Officials in Arkansas have countered these arguments by suggesting that the BMI is merely a tool. They encourage parents to seek confirmation from their family physician and argue that the goal of Act 1220 is to provide parents with important facts and confirm that weight problems are on the rise.[41]

INTERVENING TO HELP OBESE AND OVERWEIGHT STUDENTS BY SIMPLY ADVISING THEM TO CONSULT WITH A FAMILY PHYSICIAN OFTEN LEADS TO A DEAD END

According to Martha Raffaele, Dr. Reginald Washington, a Denver pediatrician who cochairs the American Academy of Pediatrics committee on obesity suggests that recommending doctor visits for overweight and obese students is a simple solution. "If you're a general practitioner, you see patients probably every ten minutes. It takes an hour of counseling and evaluation to even begin to do something about obesity."[42] Susan Okie, MD, author of *Fed Up! Winning the War Against Childhood Obesity*, indicates that many doctors are reluctant to confront the problem of overweight kids. Okie says that getting into the issue with families is delicate and time-consuming. It's a sensitive subject requiring tact, a detailed discussion about the child's and family's eating habits and activity levels, and plenty of parent education. The doctor needs to teach parents strategies to address the child's weight problems other than just putting the child on a diet, a frequent parental response that can be counterproductive and even harmful. It is virtually impossible to pack all the necessary questions and information into a well-child visit, which is typically a fifteen- or twenty-minute checkup that includes a physical examination, immunizations, and brief counseling about a variety of other topics.[43]

Okie points out that obesity in children or adults currently is not a reimbursable diagnosis until obesity has become severe enough to cause a medical illness. In addition, Okie indicates that physicians have traditionally received little nutrition education or training in how to assess a growing child's caloric needs or how to counsel the mother or father of an obese patient. Okie concludes that considering these disincentives, it is little wonder that doctors and other health-care providers often do not address excess weight adequately in children and may not even record it as a problem in the medical record. An even worse scenario is advising parents who have no health insurance or access to a family physician.[44]

Still I believe that well-intentioned efforts such as Pennsylvania's screening for obesity and the program's plan to send parents a letter encouraging them to share the screening information with their family doctors are a good beginning. Dr. Okie indicates that some school districts, concerned about the obesity epidemic, have decided not to rely only on doctors to alert parents whose children are overweight. Instead they are sending home health and fitness report cards, nicknamed "fat letters" by some critics.[45]

A study of one such effort in Cambridge, Massachusetts, found that among parents who received such letters, 42% of those with overweight children reported efforts to boost their children's physical activity level, 25% said they would consult the child's doctor, and 19% said they planned to put the child on a diet. Among parents of overweight children who did not receive such reports, only 13% reported plans to take any of these steps. Okie indicates that the Cambridge study also suggests that one of the pitfalls of informing parents that they have an overweight child is not giving them much guidance about what to do next. The study's authors were pleased about parents planning to encourage physical activity or consulting their child's doctor but were upset that almost one fifth said they intended to try to control their child's weight through dieting, using education materials sent home on limiting children's TV time, encouraging an hour of physical activity each day, and trying to make sure that children got at least five daily servings of fruit and vegetables. These materials also specifically discouraged parents from trying to place their overweight child on a restrictive diet, an approach that various studies have shown can actually be counterproductive. Okie indicates that unsupervised, do-it-yourself diets are not a safe or healthy option for children or adolescents. She reports a recent three-year study at Harvard Medical School that found that boys and girls who were frequent dieters gained more weight annually than those who never dieted and were also more likely to become binge eaters.[46]

A related study by researchers Birch and Fisher reported that young children whose mothers restricted their eating were more likely than other children to be overweight. Okie reminds parents that they do need to monitor their children's eating patterns, but those who focus obsessively and critically on a child's weight or eating may do considerable harm.[47] Therefore, when schools send out letters and report cards on weight, it is critical that they follow up with a variety of school- and community-based intervention resources that can offer ongoing support, information, monitoring, and referrals when needed. They must take a "we are in this together" approach rather than leaving it to parents to figure out what to do next.

THE EARLY BIRD INTERVENTION PROGRAM IN THE UNITED KINGDOM IS AN EXAMPLE OF HOW SCHOOLS CAN ACCELERATE THEIR INTERVENTION TO OVERWEIGHT AND OBESE TEENS

As I suggest, overweight and obese teens need more than a referral letter from their schools. In addition to a referral to a family physician, obese students such as Dylan need a school-based multipronged approach to effect major change, an approach that involves a number of school- and community-based resources that have the opportunity and, as Dr. Washington suggests, the time, for counseling of students in intervention; monitoring of their weight, diet, and related health risks such as smoking, diabetes, and so forth; an ongoing regimen of rigorous physical activity; opportunities to share their successes in losing weight and becoming sources of information and hope for their peers; support when they relapse; counseling and support for other family members; and outreach to family physicians and mental and medical health resources in the community.

One example is the Early Bird Intervention research and intervention program in the United Kingdom. This study, sponsored by the British National Institute for Diabetes and Digestive and Kidney Disease, started in 2000 to follow 300 randomly selected children and their families for twelve years. In the study, eighth-grade students with an average age of 13.6 years were asked to report to school in the morning in a fasting state and have their height, weight, waist circumference, and blood pressure, among other parameters, measured as well as having blood drawn for analysis of glucose levels, insulin, and cholesterol.

The study found that 49.3% of the children had a BMI above the eighty-fifth percentile for their age and gender. Further, 40.2% had prediabetes. Some early cases of diabetes, hypertension, and elevated cholesterol were also found in these eighth-grade students. Alison N. Jeffrey, senior research nurse on the Early Bird Survey at Demford Hospital, Peninsula Medical School, Plymouth, United Kingdom, said the results of this research effort will lead to implementing a three-year program that will assess the school environment in nutrition and physical activity and generate behavior changes in students in those areas outside of school as well.[48]

Simply put, letters to parents who are obese themselves and who do not perceive themselves or their children to be at risk of health problems caused by poor diet and lack of regular physical activity can be a wasted effort on the part of schools. Letters to parents of obese students who have normal weights themselves will not fare much better. In my counseling experience I have found that many parents of obese children are simply unaware that their children's weight is above normal. If schools are serious about the health risks for overweight and obese students, what is required is direct, face-to-face intervention with parents. In my experience, parent motivation and responsibility to act to change increase dramatically when ongoing intervention, information, monitoring, and support by the school are present. An arena of comfort is needed for parents like Margo, one that provides them with a respite and time to begin re-organizing their lives. The burden of change no longer becomes simply a "personal responsibility" effort for the parents or child. Instead it is a shared effort, a wellness pyramid, with the family, school, and community resources. That requires, as the *Breaking Ranks II: Strategies for Leading High School Reform* report recommends, that "the school leadership team successfully interact with 'hard to reach' parents with activities such as home visits, Saturday meetings and meetings outside the regular school hours."[49]

PEER INFLUENCE CAN BE A MAJOR FACTOR IN HELPING OVERWEIGHT AND OBESE TEENS ADOPT A HEALTHIER LIFESTYLE

The *National Research Newsletter* suggests that the diets of most adolescents are not consistent with the U.S. dietary guidelines. Peer-led initiatives offer a promising approach for encouraging behavioral changes among adolescents. Studies have shown that they improve young people's self-esteem, self-efficacy, knowledge, and attitudes.[50] The *Trying Alternative Cafeteria Options in Schools* study was developed to increase the number of lower-fat foods available in à la carte lines and vending machines and to increase sales of these foods in high schools during 2000 to 2002. Student-led promotional activities were incorporated into the intervention schools. Students in the ten intervention schools who participated were classified into two groups. Highly involved students were defined as those who volunteered to participate as part of extracurricular activities, internships, or independent class projects. Less-involved students were defined as those who participated because their teachers were implementing the activities as part of the curriculum. Each group of students filled out a survey that assessed their perceptions of eating behaviors, attitudes, and social norms related to lower-fat foods and perceived benefits and experiences from being involved in the project.[51]

The result of the intervention revealed a high percentage of both highly involved and less-involved students reporting that the program helped them to recognize which foods were lower in fat and that they perceived more students eating lower-fat foods in the school cafeteria since the beginning of the research project. While the highly involved students were more likely to report healthful eating behaviors and positive attitudes toward lower-fat foods than less involved students, the majority of both groups reported that student involvement was important in changing the way adolescents eat and resulted in more students trying lower-fat foods. According to the *National Research Newsletter*, the data indicate that youth may prefer to deliver health education themselves and to receive it from their peers.[52]

PARENTS AND TEACHERS CAN PLAY AN IMPORTANT MODELING ROLE IN HELPING TEENS LOSE WEIGHT

As researcher Leonard H. Epstein and colleagues suggest, in management of obesity in children it is important to consider the behavioral issues that can be used to the best advantage in family-based treatment and can best promote joint parent-child change. Epstein and colleagues cite three sets of factors to consider. First, modeling allows parents to make changes that set the stage for changes in the child. Second, parents can promote new, healthier behaviors by altering the home environment, for example, by not storing high-calorie food in the house and limiting access to television viewing. Third, the inclusion of both parents and children in the treatment produces the opportunity for joint reinforcement of a change in habits. Parents can be trained to reinforce new behaviors, and the children can do the same for parents.[53]

As in Dylan's case, efforts to involve Margo, Kyle, and Kate in developing an intervention plan for a healthier lifestyle sets the stage for Margo to begin modeling such a lifestyle for her children and for Dylan to begin using his newly learned health-promoting skills for Kyle, Kate, and Margo. The intervention plan calls for educators—such as assistant principal Al Morris, nutritionist Nancy Clifford, nurse Barbara Grant, counselor Brad Langdon, physical education teachers Tony Jankowski and Marge Edgar, and homeroom teacher/advisor Martha Mayer—to model a variety of healthy lifestyles that can assist Dylan in making necessary behavioral changes.

COMPASSIONATE TREATMENT IS A MAJOR FACTOR IN HELPING OVERWEIGHT AND OBESE TEENS TO DEVELOP HEALTHY LIFESTYLES AND LOSE WEIGHT

As researchers Thomas A. Wadden and Barbara J. Wingate advise, it is hard to imagine the prejudice and discrimination that overweight individuals endure. Nasty remarks can be found even in our nation's respected newsweeklies. As quoted by Wadden and Wingate, the author of a "My Turn" column in *Newsweek* wrote, "This information [about genetic determinants of obesity] should be withheld from the fat multitudes because the obese will latch onto any excuse for failing to lose weight. Face it, Chubbo, when was the last time you were force-fed?" According to Wadden and Wingate, these sentiments illustrate all too clearly that obesity is still regarded by laypersons, and many practitioners, as a moral rather than a medical problem. It is attributed to indulgence, lack of willpower, and similar failings, accusations that allow lean individuals to feel morally superior.[54]

Regrettably, many overweight individuals have internalized this view at the expense of their self-esteem and self-respect. Dylan's daily bout with himself as he looks into the mirror each morning and says, "What a fat shit! Look at me! I am revolting," gives us a flavor of the cost to teens when they internalize their weight problems. Wadden and Wingate's research suggests that for most overweight individuals, efforts to lose weight often exacerbate rather than heal their psychological injuries. A small percentage enjoy weight control, but the great majority feel shame, frustration, and humiliation as they lose and regain weight in full view of family, friends, healthcare providers, and, in the case of teens, their peers and teachers. Most dieters blame themselves for their lack of weight loss and inability to control their weight.[55]

Wadden and Wingate argue that what is needed in intervention to help individuals lose weight is respect and concern, some effort to reduce weight-related stress.[56] In my experience counseling overweight and obese teens, that means understanding the frustration and disappointment of students like Dylan in dealing with their weight. I have found that understanding comes with listening to their stories about being overweight or obese, asking them to write about their experiences, and, in support groups, asking them to act out the prejudice and discrimination they have endured as overweight children and adolescents. It is a process that requires educators to walk in their shoes and experience the daily bouts that have long been a part of the lives of teens like Dylan, and to be compassionate—to have the ability and skills to sympathize deeply, accompanied by a wish to help. Little successes—a two-pound weight loss, a forty-minute workout, lowered blood pressure, a week without pizza, enrolling in a school nutrition program, cutting back on tobacco smoking and alcohol on weekends, encouraging a parent to enroll in evening nutrition workshops, and so forth—can provide an "I can do this" foundation, energy, and the strength needed as they face resistance from themselves, peers, and parents.

In my counseling experience with overweight and obese teens, I have found that one of the most difficult problems they face is overcoming the resistance they face from obese parents, peers, and themselves. Some parents will counter a teen's goal to lose weight with comments like, "You are fine. The family is a little heavy, but what's wrong with that? Tell those school people to stick to teaching and stop poking into your weight and our family business. If you won't tell them, I will." Some obese peers will challenge with remarks like, "I see you've begun attending nurse Grant and counselor Langdon's groups. What's the deal? Our group's no longer good enough for you? Next thing you'll be giving up smoking and become one of those phony do-good peer counselors." Obese teens like Dylan, who have internalized all the hurts and put-downs, may feel that they are not worthy of change, that they are indeed "fat shits, slobs, chubbos" and that they don't deserve to be anything different. Compassionate educators can make a huge difference in advising students like Dylan how to successfully navigate around these assaults and overcome family and peer resistance as well as their own resistance to fit in and become part of the school community.

By modeling, listening, challenging, supporting, and reinforcing overweight and obese students, compassionate educators can help them come to believe that they are no longer sentenced to the margins of school life, where all they can do is observe the happiness, success, and rewards of other students. They have the opportunity and support to come out of the obese closet, take their place, and walk confidently down the hallways, no longer afraid to be called names, bullied, pushed around, and made to believe they are simply "fat shits" and "chubbos" whose only existence and value to the school is to be the target of others' hostility.

SCHOOL- AND COMMUNITY-BASED REMEDIES TO HELP TEENS LOSE WEIGHT ARE DOABLE AND NOT COMPLICATED

I believe Beth Trapani, spokeswoman for the Pennsylvania Advocates for Nutrition and Activity, the group that is helping the Pennsylvania

State Health Department publicize the BMI screening in the schools, is right on target when she suggests that remedies for child and teen weight loss are doable and not complicated. The School Nutrition Association, in conjunction with the National School Lunch Week program, awarded Preston High School in the Bronx, New York, a $15,000 grant to help fund the school's physical activity program. The school stresses the importance of both good nutrition, including the recent addition of a salad bar to the cafeteria, and physical activity through the student fitness program, "Fun-n-Fitness," that the school recently developed. The "Fun-n-Fitness" program includes classes that involve stretching, toning, aerobics, free-weight training, dietary information, and an after-school walking program.[57]

The National School Lunch Week program is designed to raise awareness of the importance that school nutrition plays in the lives of American children.[58] As researcher Dr. Jennifer Zebrack advises, "Little things add up for teens who want to lose weight."[59] Preston High provides a useful example of the uncomplicated remedies schools can implement—a salad bar in the cafeteria, a "Fun-n-Fitness" program, dietary information, and an after-school walking program—that might also include a before-school and lunchtime walking component.[60]

I have also personally experienced the value of uncomplicated remedies in efforts to improve teens' well-being as an education reformer helping to develop the Louis Armstrong Intermediate School in Queens, New York. In an effort to attract students and parents to enroll at Louis Armstrong, the leadership team from Queens College introduced a number of programs to help improve the well-being and academics of students and education opportunities for parents: a before-school "Early Bird" breakfast and tutorial program, an after-school tutorial and physical activity program, a summer physical activity program that included breakfast and lunch, a mentorship program for teachers to advise students on academic, personal, health, and well-being issues, and evening and weekend workshops on parenting, health issues, and education/training opportunities that involved Queens College staff and resources. These were all uncomplicated remedies that called for the school to be open from 7:00 A.M. to 9:00 P.M. and on weekends.

The Preston High School and Louis Armstrong Intermediate
School interventions are examples of a growing number of innovative
programs in our schools that focus on improving students' nutrition
and increasing physical activity levels. A key component in the success of these programs is the leadership and modeling of administrators, such as Moorhead's Al Morris, who send a clear signal to professional and support staff, students, and parents that students
afflicted by health and well-being problems such as obesity matter
and need caring and helpful intervention from every member of the
school community. As the American Obesity Association points out,
parents want changes in the schools' nutrition and physical activity
programs. The association reports that 36% of parents rated their
children's school programs for teaching good patterns of eating and
physical activity as "poor," "non-existent," or "don't know." A majority of parents in the United States (78%) believe physical education
or recess should not be reduced or replaced with academic classes.[61]

I believe changes in the nutrition and physical activity programs
in the schools will come about only when educators understand the
health risks for overweight and obese students, as I have described
in this chapter, and also the unique opportunity they have to direct
students to sources of help and education in the school and community and model a healthy lifestyle. The report *Preventing Childhood Obesity: Health in the Balance* states that schools are one of the
primary locations for reaching the nation's children and youth. In
2000, 53.2 million students were enrolled in public and private elementary and secondary schools in the United States. Both inside
and outside the classroom, schools present opportunities for students to learn about good nutrition, physical activity, and their relationship to health; to engage in physical education; and to make food
and physical activity choices during school mealtimes and through
school-related activities.[62]

The next chapter will focus on how school mealtimes can be improved in order to help students learn about good nutrition and
make healthy food choices. Understanding obesity is the first step in
developing an intervention process, a first step that must be followed by direct, concrete, visible action.

NOTES

1. Mike Smith, "More High School Students Overweight; Drug Use, Smoking Down," Associated Press, 18 Oct. 2005, http://www2.indystar.com/articles/0/241135-9530-P.html (accessed 25 Oct. 2005).

2. Smith, "More High School Students Overweight."

3. Empire Plan, "Considering the Cost of Obesity," *Taking Care: Helping People Stay Healthy Since 1978*, vol. 27, no. 9 (September 2004): 8.

4. Michael D. Lemonick, "How We Grew So Big," *Time Magazine/ABC News Report*, "America's Obesity Crisis," 7 June 2004, 1–7.

5. Jeffrey Kluger, Christine Gorman, and Alice Park, "Why We Eat," *Time Magazine/ABC News Report*, "America's Obesity Crisis," 7 June 2004, 8–11.

6. Claudia Wallis, "The Obesity Warriors," *Time Magazine/ABC News Report*, "America's Obesity Crisis," 7 June 2004, 12–16.

7. ChiroTips.com, "How to Get Fat Without Really Trying," summary of ABC News broadcast of 8 Dec. 2003, http://www.chirotips.com/how_to_get_fat_without_really_tr.htm (accessed 6 June 2005).

8. Kaiser Family Foundation, "Report on Role of Media in Childhood Obesity," Kaiser Family Foundation, 24 Feb. 2004, http://www.kff.org/entmedia/entmedia022404nr.cfm?RenderForPrint=1 (accessed 25 May 2005).

9. Medical College of Wisconsin (MCI) Health News, "U.S. Obesity at an All-Time High," HealthLink, 26 Nov. 2002, http://healthlink.mcw.edu/articles/1031002183.html (accessed 22 June 2005).

10. Gary Ruskin, "The Fast Food Trap: How Commercialism Creates Overweight Children," *Mothering*, no. 121, Nov.–Dec. 2003, http://www.commercialalert.org/index.php/categlory_id/5.subcategory_id/72/article_id/236 (accessed 25 May 2005).

11. Joy Johanson, "Nutrition Integrity in Schools," Center for Science in the Public Interest, 2004, http://www.cspinet.org/nutritionpolicy.fedschoolfoods.pdf (accessed 4 Apr. 2005).

12. C. B. Ebberling, K. B. Sinclair, M.A. Pereira, et al., "Compensation for Energy Intake From Fast Food Among Overweight and Lean Adolescents," American Diabetes Association, 2004, http://www.diabetes.org/utils/printthispage.jsp?PageID=RESEARCHRESOURCES_288154 (accessed 24 May 2005).

13. J. A. Welsh, M. E. Cogswell, S. Rogers, et al., "Overweight Among Low-Income Preschool Children Associated with the Consumption of Sweet Drinks; Missouri, 1999–2002," American Diabetes Association, 2004,

http://www.diabetes.org/utils/printthispage.jsp?PageID=RESEARCHRE
SOURCES_288638 (accessed 24 May 2005).

14. S. A. Bowman and B. T. Vinyard, "Fast-Food Consumption of U.S. Adults: Impact on Energy and Nutrient Intake and Overweight Status," American Diabetes Association, 2004, http://www.diabetes.org/utils/print thispage.jsp?PageID=researchresources_287685 (accessed 24 May 2005).

15. Welsh, Cogswell, Rogers, et al., "Overweight Among Low-Income Preschool Children."

16. School Nutrition Association, "California Teens Fixed on Junk Food," *Contra Costa (CA) Times*, 13 Sept. 2005, http://www.schoolnutrition.org/ Article.aspx?SMDOCID=krdigital_2005_09_13_eng-krdig (accessed 13 Oct. 2005).

17. School Nutrition Association, "California Teens Fixed on Junk Food."

18. ABC News, "Nightline: Critical Condition–Obesity Crisis," 2 June 2004, abcNEWSstore.com, http://www.abcnewsstore.com/store/index.cfm? fuseaction+customer.product&product_cod (accessed 31 May 2005).

19. School Nutrition Association, "California Teens Fixed on Junk Food."

20. E. D. Hirsch Jr., *The Schools We Need* (New York: Doubleday, 1996), 33–55.

21. Geneva Gay, *Culturally Responsive Teaching* (New York: Teachers College Press, 2000), vi, 17–19, 45–46.

22. Stephanie Rosenbloom, "Fat, O.K.? And Having a Blast," *New York Times*, 23 June 2005, G1–2.

23. Kluger, Gorman, and Park, "Why We Eat," 8–11.

24. Jeffrey B. Schwimmer, "Child Obesity Hurts Emotional Health," *Education Week Health Update*, 23 April 2003, http://www.edweek.org/ew/ articles/2004/04/23/32health.h22.html?print=1 (accessed 25 May 2005).

25. J. Williams, M. Wake, K. Hesbeth, et al., "Health-related Quality of Life of Overweight and Obese Children," American Diabetes Association, 2005, http://www.diabetes.org/utils/printthispage.jsp?PageID=RESEARCH RESOURCES_290662 (accessed 24 May 2005).

26. Abby Ellin, "For Overweight Children, Are 'Fat Camps' a Solution?" *New York Times*, 28 June 2005, F1, F8.

27. Lindsey Tanner, "Suicide Attempts Linked to Weight Perception," boston.com, 7 June 2005, http://www.boston.com/yourlife/health/ children/articles/2005/06/07/suicide_attempts_link (accessed 12 June 2005).

28. William H. Dietz, "Health Consequences of Obesity in Youth: Childhood Predictors of Adult Diseases," *Pediatrics 101*, no. 3 (March 1998): 518–21.

29. Marsha D. Marcus, "Binge Eating and Obesity," in *Binge Eating: Nature, Assessment, and Treatment*, ed. Christopher G. Fairburn and G. Terrence Wilson (New York: Guilford Press, 1993), 77–96.

30. Raja Mishra, "Adult Diabetes Hitting Children," boston.com, 12 June 2005, http://www.boston.com/yourlife/health/children/articles/2005.06/12/adult_diabetes_hitting (accessed 12 June 2005).

31. Jane E. Brody, "'Diabesity,' a Crisis in an Expanding Country," *New York Times*, 29 Mar. 2005, F8.

32. Brody, "'Diabesity,'" F8.

33. Brody, "'Diabesity,'" F8.

34. Lisa Sanders, "Diagnosis," *New York Times Magazine*, 21 Sept. 2003, sec. 6, p. 24.

35. Martha Raffaele, "Pa. Screening Schoolchildren for Obesity," Associated Press, 14 Sept. 2005, http://www.yahoo.com/s/ap/20050914/ap_on_he_me/fit_weighing_schoolchildren_2 (accessed 15 Sept. 2005).

36. Roni Rabin, "Built Just for Kids," *Newsday*, 29 Sept. 2005, A4.

37. Marianne D. Hurst, "Arkansas Pupils' Body Weights Add Up," *Education Week*, 15 Sept. 2004, http://www.edweek.org/ew/articles/2004.09/15.03bmi,h24.html?print=1 (accessed 25 May 2005).

38. Hurst, "Arkansas Pupils' Body Weights."

39. Sally Squires, "One Number Doesn't Fit All," *Washington Post*, 5 July 2005, http://www.washingtonpost.com/wp-dyn/content/articles/2005/07/04/AR2005070400949_pf (accessed 6 July 2005).

40. American Enterprise Institute (AEI), "Obesity, Individual Responsibility, and Public Policy," *AEI Newsletter*, 23 July 2003, http://www.aei.org/publications/pubID.18073,filter.economic/pub_detail.asp (accessed 22 June 2005).

41. Hurst, "Arkansas Pupils' Body Weights."

42. Raffaele, "Pa. Screening Schoolchildren."

43. Susan Okie, *Fed Up! Winning the War Against Childhood Obesity* (Washington, DC: Joseph Henry Press, 2005), 59–60.

44. Okie, *Fed Up!* 59–60.

45. Okie, *Fed Up!* 62–63.

46. Okie, *Fed Up!* 62–63.

47. Okie, *Fed Up!* 57–66.

48. American Diabetes Association, "Overweight Families Unaware & Unconcerned—Then Diabetes Hits Kids," American Diabetes Association press release, 4 June 2004, http://www.diabetes.org/for-media/2004-press-releases/overweight-families.jsp (accessed 24 May 2005).

49. National Association of Secondary School Principals (NASSP), *Executive Summary of Breaking Ranks II: Strategies for Leading High School Reform* (Reston, VA: NASSP, 2004), 1–6.

50. National Research Newsletter, "Adolescent Involvement in Nutrition Programs," *LookSmart,* March 2005, http://www.findarticles.com/p/articles/mi_m0887/is_3_24/ai_n13648424/print (accessed 23 Oct. 2005).

51. National Research Newsletter, "Adolescent Involvement."

52. National Research Newsletter, "Adolescent Involvement."

53. Leonard H. Epstein et al., "Ten Year Follow-up of Behavioral, Family-based Treatment for Obese Children," *Journal of the American Medical Association* 264 (1990): 2519–23.

54. Thomas A. Wadden and Barbara J. Wingate, "Compassionate Treatment of the Obese Individual," in *Binge Eating: Nature, Assessment, and Treatment,* ed. Christopher G. Fairburn and G. Terrence Wilson (New York: Guilford Press, 1993), 564–71.

55. Wadden and Wingate, "Compassionate Treatment," 564–68.

56. Wadden and Wingate, "Compassionate Treatment," 568–71.

57. School Nutrition Association, "Bronx HS Rewarded in Healthy Schools Challenge," School Nutrition Association press release, 2005, http://www.schoolnutrition.org/PrinterFriendly.aspx>id=1643 (accessed 27 Oct. 2005).

58. School Nutrition Association, "Bronx HS Rewarded."

59. Medical College of Wisconsin (MCI) Health News, "U.S. Obesity."

60. School Nutrition Association, "Bronx HS Rewarded."

61. American Obesity Association, "Finally a Cure for Obesity," American Obesity Association press release, 2002, http://obesity.org/subs/childhood/prevention.shtml (accessed 25 May 2005).

62. Jeffrey P. Kaplan, Catharyn T. Liverman, and Vivica I. Kraak, editors, *Preventing Childhood Obesity: Health in the Balance* (Washington, DC: National Academies Press, 2004), 237.

4

HOW SCHOOL WELLNESS COUNCILS CAN REVITALIZE THE CAFETERIA AND FOOD SERVICE SYSTEM

Savvy administrators such as Moorhead High's Al Morris understand that the effort to provide students with healthy food alternatives to the fast-food restaurants surrounding many large high schools begins with redesigning the school cafeteria, elevating the cafeteria food delivery system to a centerpiece in the school's health and wellness intervention program. The process can transform an aged relic into a welcoming and attractive setting where students want to be, a learning laboratory for students on how to develop healthy eating habits, and, for staff, a research laboratory focused on what works to win students over to healthy nutrition. It will become a setting that sends the message that the school is serious about making sure students have healthy food options. Such a centerpiece cafeteria might offer the following:

- An attractive buffet menu throughout the school day, featuring natural juices, fruits, cereals, vegetables, grains, cheese, and low-fat milk products. It can also include pizza, pasta, breads, and burgers made with healthy ingredients to satisfy the fast-food crowd.
- A warm and courteous service team who receive regular training on how to relate to and understand adolescents, present

welcoming and caring role models, and receive ongoing positive feedback regarding their value and worth in improving the overall school climate

- A decor that teens can relate to, such as festive pictures, posters, colorful chairs and tables, a computer lounge, and music playing in the background
- The opportunity for meaningful student-adult communication by serving faculty, support staff, and students together as part of the school community
- The opportunity for students like Dylan to attend short-term workshops led by cafeteria dietitians and food service workers on low-fat meal preparation, changing eating habits, shopping wisely for food, eating healthy on a minimum budget, making sense of health messages from the media, and so forth
- A Nutritional and Health Information Center that provides information on health and wellness, adolescent health problems, nutrition, weight reduction, drug and alcohol abuse, tobacco use, self-help, intervention for family members and peers, Internet health and wellness resources, and family and personal counseling services offered in the community
- An on-site resource room manned before school, during each class period, and after school by a member of the school's intervention team and community health and counseling professionals. These might include a counselor, physical education teachers, the school nurse, a health teacher, and representatives from community health agencies. It can be a setting that offers daily health and well-being workshops, screening for blood pressure, and referral information, a program that brings information and support directly to students in their territory rather than their having to go to an outside office for help. In my experience with teens, offering health and wellness support and information on their own ground has a greater potential for success. In the minds of many teenagers, offices, even when manned by the best of caring professionals, still carry the negative connotation of places where troubled teens end up and are therefore places to be avoided.

- A weekly health and nutrition e-mail newsletter sent to interested students, which offers monthly online chat sessions where students can share health and nutrition information, tips on how to develop healthy habits, hints to improve overall health, and resources that appear to aid students' behavioral changes
- The opportunity for students to take leadership roles as members of the school's wellness council, which oversees the food service system, and also to be employed as part-time members of the cafeteria staff
- Easily accessible opportunities for students to provide feedback on food service, such as online evaluation forms and suggestion boxes

It will be a setting that offers a respite from the pressures of schooling, nutritious food to help students maintain a high level of energy, the opportunity to communicate with peers and staff, and health and wellness information and referrals when needed. Teens will eat healthy foods if they are available in a cafeteria setting where the teens are welcomed, where their presence is valued, where they will be missed if they are absent, and where they can laugh and interact with peers and faculty.

The setting I am describing here is no fantasy. Many corporations are creating the same kind of food service ambience for their workers. They offer an option to encourage workers to change their eating patterns by choosing to eat on-site rather than partake of unhealthy food and drink at restaurants. This option is part of a broader wellness program that includes daily opportunities for physical fitness, workshops on health and wellness issues, regular monitoring of key health indicators such as blood pressure, cholesterol, blood sugar levels, and so forth, and opportunities for counseling intervention to address issues such as the relationship between health and absences from work. These companies offer a place that helps workers get away from the pressures of their workday, communicate with peers and management, eat attractive and nourishing foods, have the opportunity to take part in health and wellness workshops, and have access to community health and counseling resources. Workers get a mealtime break, a healthy pause that readies them to return to challenges of the workplace. *OC Metro*, a business lifestyle magazine, suggests that about 50% of companies have some type of employee wellness program in place, programs in which senior management makes tackling health problems such as obesity a business priority.[1] I believe schools can provide the same kind of high-quality wellness and food service by embracing this corporate model.

Here is a step-by-step plan that administrators can follow to revitalize their school cafeterias and make them competitive and a teaching model for healthy eating:

CREATE A PLAN FOR A REVITALIZED FOOD SERVICE THAT PLACES THE SCHOOL CAFETERIA AT THE CENTER OF A BROADER SCHOOL WELLNESS PROGRAM BASED ON A CORPORATE WELLNESS MODEL

In developing a plan to revitalize the school food service system, I encourage administrators to conceptualize the school cafeteria as one of the essential building blocks needed to address the health issues of students and staff, such as being overweight and obese. I argue that the role of the cafeteria needs to be elevated from simply a place where some students gather to hang out and eat to a place in which the cafeteria plays a major role in the school's intervention plan, that is, joining other school health and counseling services to provide blood pressure screening, blood sugar and cholesterol screening, alcohol and drug abuse prevention, eating disorder intervention, smoking cessation, rigorous physical activity, health and wellness education, parent education, and easy access to community health and counseling services.

Many corporations offer similar wellness services to their workers in order to reduce absenteeism, improve workers' health, increase awareness of wellness issues, reduce overall health costs, promote a healthy work climate, and increase productivity. I believe these corporate wellness models can serve the same positive function for students by reducing absenteeism, dealing with acting-out behaviors such as bullying, teaching students how to develop a healthier lifestyle, helping students become aware of health risks associated with overweight and obesity and how to avoid such risks, providing early intervention before such problems arise, increasing awareness of wellness issues, making students aware of sources of support in the school and community, and increasing students' productivity.

There are many parallels between workers and students. Workers spend many of their waking hours at work, and therefore food eaten at work contributes significantly to their total daily intake. Most employees will eat at work nearly every workday, which provides the opportunity for regular nutrition education and access to information/intervention in the workplace cafeteria. The same can be said for students.

In my research for this book I found that many high school administrators are beginning to grasp the concept of a school-wide health and wellness effort to modify adverse health risks to students, an effort that requires the many individual educators involved in offering health and counseling support, often separated and isolated from each other, to become part of a team effort with each member—counselor, nurse, dietitian, physical education teacher, student assistance counselor, health teacher—making a unique and special contribution. Some administrators have observed that schools can successfully intervene to help students with alcohol, drug, and tobacco addictions, family violence, and poor peer relationships, such as bullying.

This kind of intervention model can also be used to address the related health and well-being issues of students. Some future-oriented administrators are also beginning to grasp that the school's wellness effort needs to include addressing the health and well-being issues of staff. "Look, we have staff who are overweight, obese, heavy smokers, alcoholics, bulimic, anorexic, and so on. You name it and we have it right here. These issues are killing us with absenteeism, staff turnover, unprofessional behaviors, students and parents avoiding some teachers, and so forth. We have to bring these issues out of the closet so these guys and gals get the help they need. It's way beyond being just a supervision problem. I'm hoping our new wellness team will begin offering the same kinds of support and intervention to staff that the kids get. We can't continue to ignore the health and well-being risks for educators who are involved each day with students and parents. We need to be promoting the notion that we can't allow any member of our school community to slip through the cracks, not just our students."

In the end we need programs and policies in the schools that make the health of every member of the school community—students, parents, support staff, faculty, and administrators—a high priority. As part of that process, the newly mandated wellness councils in each school need to keep in mind that eating well and being physically active take more than just willpower. Easily accessible open doors for help need to be made clear and welcoming for students like Dylan. And school administrators need to make tackling health issues such as obesity a high priority, just as many leaders of corporations do.

BE REALISTIC: IN THE BEGINNING, SET YOUR GOAL TO REACH A PERCENTAGE OF STUDENTS

As Al Morris understands, it is politically unwise to abruptly make major changes in student eating policies, such as moving from an open to a closed campus, even if these policies are based on good intentions. As I suggested in chapter 2, abrupt changes in policies often result in student and parent resistance and hardened positions that can lead to standoffs and prolonged negotiations. Instead, I would advise administrators to try to reach a middle ground with students and parents by offering a competitive food service in the school that can serve to lure a percentage of students back to campus for mealtime. I urge administrators and faculty leaders to try to win over the hearts, minds, and stomachs of students by putting their energy and resources into creating attractive in-school eating options.

IN THE EFFORT TO REVITALIZE THE CAFETERIA FOOD SERVICE SYSTEM, ADMINISTRATORS NEED TO DEVELOP A PLAN THAT FOCUSES ON THE PARTICULAR NEEDS OF STUDENTS AND STAFF IN THEIR SCHOOL AND UTILIZE THEIR OWN SCHOOL-BASED WELLNESS TEAM TO SPEARHEAD SUCH AN EFFORT; SUCCESSFUL REFORM EFFORTS NEED TO BE SUPPORTED AT THE BUILDING LEVEL

As I have suggested, many corporate wellness programs are successful because company leaders have make tackling workers' health issues a business priority. In my experience I have found building principals, with the support of the superintendent and the school board, to be the key players in spearheading this kind of educational reform. Why? Building principals know their staff, students, and parents, and they understand what needs to be done to sell education reform such as a wellness program. They know how to get various members of the school community on board the project; face and overcome staff, parent, community, and even student resistance; gather together a broad section of staff to help lead the step-by-step implementation process; be flexible and able to change directions when failure arises; and, finally, highlight the project's successes and its value to staff, students, parents, and community members.

I have found that a building-based reform process led by the principal, with strong faculty support, has a much greater chance for success than a district-wide reform effort led by the superintendent and including building principals and staff from each school in the district. Why? Every school has its own special culture and needs. Principals and faculty in each district school often have little understanding of what goes on in other buildings. They rarely if ever visit other schools and observe how the education process works. Principals and faculty may belong to one school district, but the reality is that they spend most of their careers in one building. The result is that when these principals and faculty are asked to serve on district-wide policy committees to implement education reform mandates from state or federal agencies, the process often moves at a snail's pace. It takes members time to get to know each other and learn what will be the impact of the reform, what changes it will bring to their building and turf, who will be the winners and have more political clout in the anticipated change, and who will be the losers. There is a lot of jockeying in education reform committees, subtle infighting between elementary and secondary staff members, and building resistance when their turf is threatened. In my experience, not much is accomplished, and members leave feeling lured into another education reform that never succeeds.

I have been part of such a scenario as founder and director of the Bay Shore Public Schools/Stony Brook University Teacher Center, a school-day teacher training program led by teachers for their peers with financial support from a nearby university. This unique project began as a staff-led effort following a staff development workshop that focused on how to improve school climate for the over 200 staff members and 2,000 students from a variety of ethnic and cultural backgrounds. The building principal, like Al Morris, was quick to grasp the value of the "teachers training teachers" concept and the resources available to the school from Stony Brook University. Empowering staff to train their peers in new curriculum, discipline, and advising approaches was a key component.

After early resistance, over 90% of the staff eventually became involved as trainers in daily workshops offered during staff free periods and mealtime. Staff members were won over by a process of ongoing invitations to come aboard the project even after they voiced strong verbal resistance. The project became a success. Staff morale rose, discipline problems were reduced, staff came to understand the many resources they had in fellow teachers, and parents and community members became more connected to the school. The project attracted educators from local, state, national, and international schools. We had a winning formula for education reform at Bay Shore Junior High, with strong backing from the principal, who helped maintain the backing of the superintendent and school board.

But all that changed with the emergence of federal funding for teacher centers. The funding process required that school districts put in place a governing board, including staff and administration from each school building as well as the superintendent. It seemed a good idea at first glance. From the superintendent's view, the upside of seeking funding would mean that the teacher center would be on more permanent ground, as the district was having budget problems. Also, the center would now be able to offer training district-wide. However, there was a downside felt by the staff and principal at the junior high. They felt that the teacher center, their baby, was about to be taken from them and made a district-level program. They felt they were being sold down the river, to use a common description of betrayal. A grassroots effort begun by a cadre of teachers with the support of the principal to help improve the school climate in the junior high was about to be shifted outside their building to other district schools and staff, many of whom had no interest in the project or, as in the high school, many staff who were not about to give up their lunch time or free period to be taught by peers.

But as the reader knows, the lure of possible federal funding often wins out over such staff concerns. A district teacher center governing board was formed to seek funding. However, not only did the request for funding fail but the onset of the district's control of the center spelled the end of the vibrant teacher center at the junior high. Here is what happened and the lessons learned on my part.

The teacher center project, while still serving the junior high school, moved to the district level and had the mandate to serve the other four schools in the district. But there were dire results. The staff at the junior high was left with fewer resources, such as funds to hire substitute teachers to fill in for teachers who offered training at the center. In addition, the teacher center staff was spread thin in an effort to develop principal and staff support in the other school buildings. The result? The teacher center at the junior high slowly collapsed because the project was overextended and, most important, lost its junior high faculty support and vital political base. While I had left the district to lead staff development work in another setting, I kept in touch with the cadre of junior high staff and the principal who launched the center. They felt abandoned and betrayed by the intrusion and meddling of the district in a successful program.

I learned many lessons in this cycle of success and failure. For example, what works in one school for educational reform may not be
successful in another setting. Education reform that works often
emerges from the needs of staff to improve conditions for themselves, students, and parents and from the availability of a cadre of
leaders, including the building principal, who are willing to take the
risk to create new ways of doing business, move a good idea successfully into the school environment even when resistance is high,
and take ownership and pride in what their good idea and risks have
produced. However, when that good idea is viewed as something
every school in the district should be doing, projects like the teacher
center lose the hearts and souls of those who took the initial risk to
get on board and fail in the effort to bring in new blood from other
schools who in reality lack the roots, understanding, and ownership
in the project.

This is the kind of downside that can happen to Al Morris and his
Wellness Team, who have developed a grassroots effort to address
student health and well-being issues. His is a building-based program that focuses on the needs of students and staff at Moorhead
High, *not* the other schools in the district. Morris has managed to
bring together a talented team made up of nurse Barbara Grant, dietitian Nancy Clifford, student assistance counselor Brad Langdon,
physical education teachers Tony Jankowski and Marge Edgar, student advisors such as Martha Mayer, and Child Study Team chair
Harry Polk. They form a team that is ready and set to act when they
observe an obese student such as Dylan, a team that is focused on
the Moorhead High School community and its needs.

I argue that it is critical for administrators to keep the model of
Al Morris and Moorhead High at the forefront as they try to put in
place a district Local Wellness Policy by July 1, 2006. The policy is
mandated for all school districts that participate in the National
School Lunch Program and is part of the reauthorized Child Nutrition Act of 2004. The new law says that local policies must include
goals for nutrition education, physical activity, and nutrition guidelines selected by the local educational agency; establish a plan for
measuring implementation of the local wellness policy; and involve

parents, students, representatives of the school food authority, the school board, administrators, and the public in the development of the school wellness policy.

The Child Nutrition Act also specifically addresses the problem of childhood obesity on several fronts. The law requires that districts appoint wellness committees, which must include a variety of members, such as students, teachers, community members, and representatives of the district's food service program. The wellness plan drawn up by each committee must deal with the types of food sold in schools, physical education, and nutrition.[2] Janet Brown, program officer for the Center for Ecoliteracy, suggests that wellness committees can serve the purpose of a town meeting on wellness, with community children at the heart of the discussion. She says that, used to its fullest potential, the wellness policy development process restores authority for decisions affecting the health of children to their parents and communities. According to Brown, wellness committees do their best work when they encourage a relationship between those who work and attend school inside the district, such as students, school board members, superintendents, principals, educators, food service professionals, and school nurses, and those individuals and groups outside the school who are fully invested in the process, including parents, grandparents, and community members. The overall goal of the wellness policy is to help students be healthy, fit, and ready to learn. Brown suggests that the wellness policy requires ensuring that our children will have fresh, delicious, nutritious food every school day; a pleasant mealtime environment; sufficient time to eat; and a guarantee that opportunities for invigorating physical exercise will be available to every student every day.[3]

A Model Wellness Policy Guide produced by the Center for Ecoliteracy suggests beginning the wellness policy development process with a visionary statement of responsibility from the board of education that states, for example,

> The Board recognizes that there is a link between nutritional education, the food served in schools, [and] physical activity . . . and that wellness is affected by all of these. The Board also recognizes the

important connection between a healthy diet and a student's ability to learn effectively and achieve high standards in school. . . . The Board of Education further recognizes that the sharing and enjoyment of food, and participation in physical activities, are fundamental experiences for all people and are a primary way to nurture and celebrate our cultural diversity. These fundamental human experiences are vital bridges for building friendships, forming inter-generational bonds, and strengthening communities.

The Model Wellness Policy Guide includes suggestions on how school districts can set goals for nutrition education, physical activity, school-based learning experiences, and professional development and how schools can establish nutrition guidelines for all schools in the district. The guide also recommends that membership in the wellness committee include the superintendent, the director of child nutrition services, three support staff employees appointed by the employee organization, three teachers appointed by their employee organization, one principal appointed by the principals' employee organization, five students appointed by student government, and ten parent/community representatives appointed by the board of education.[4]

The National Alliance for Nutrition and Activity (NANA) also has developed a Model Local School Wellness Policy on Physical Activity and Nutrition that includes many of the same components of the Center for Ecoliteracy model.[5] However, the NANA wellness policy guide adds a few critical dimensions. For example, the policy uses data that are designed to sound the alarm that schools are falling short in their commitment to improve nutrition and physical activity for their students. In the preamble the policy guide states, "Thirty-three percent of high school students do not participate in sufficient vigorous physical activity and 72 percent of high school students do not attend daily physical education classes. Only two percent of children ages two through nineteen years eat a healthy diet consistent with the five main recommendations from the Food Pyramid Guide."[6]

The NANA guide uses the term "School Health Council" instead of "wellness committee." The guide also promotes the notion of staff wellness by stating the need for the school district to "highly value the health and well-being of every staff member and the need to plan and implement activities and policies that support personal efforts by staff to maintain a healthy lifestyle." The guide recommends that a staff wellness committee be established in each school and be a subcommittee of the school health council. The staff wellness committee should develop a plan to outline ways to encourage healthy eating, physical activity, and other elements of a healthy lifestyle among school staff.[7]

Like Janet Brown, I believe that the creation of local wellness policies and committees has great potential to help students be healthy, fit, and ready to learn. I applaud the NANA emphasis on staff wellness. However, I believe the well-intended Local Wellness Policy and wellness committee mandate in the reauthorized Child Nutrition Act leaves out some important components that schools need to include in order for student wellness to be reality. Here are some suggestions:

• Nowhere in the model guidelines is there a focus on the need/requirement for individual schools to have a wellness champion like Al Morris who is politically wise; is assertive; has leadership skills; can work and interact with a variety of constituents; knows and understands the needs of students, staff, and parents; has a vision of what constitutes a healthy school environment; and most important, can sell better student nutrition and physical activity to a staff and community already preoccupied, some say consumed, with raising standards while keeping budgets low. Simply put, the need is for someone who is going to lead the charge, take the heart, get the staff involved, and overcome resistance. Good ideas don't make it without "doers" like Al Morris in place. The suggestions of policy advocates such as Janet Brown, who says, "The wellness policy development supports introducing learning experiences connected to diet and health, kitchen classrooms, serving fresh seasonal locally grown food, and designing eating experiences that promote lifelong wellness,"[8] will not see the light of day in most schools without the presence of an administrator or teacher leader who can sell these ideas and projects to staff, students, parents, and community in today's rough-and-tumble school world with competing constituencies. This selling plan needs to avoid overburdening staff in the beginning stages with data that, while important, is too detailed for busy staff who want to hear only the bottom line of what the project will mean for them, their students, and their school. The NANA guidelines include recommendations for schools such as to

> serve only low-fat (1%) and fat-free milk; assure that half of the served grains are whole grains; encourage parents to provide a healthy breakfast for their children through newsletter articles, take-home material or other means . . . allow water or seltzer water without added caloric sweeteners; provide fruit and vegetable juices and fruit-based drinks that contain at least 50% fruit juice and do not contain additional caloric sweeteners, unflavored or flavored low-fat or fat-free fluid milk; and [ensure that] food items sold will have no more than 35% of [their] calories from fat and from saturated and trans-fat combined.[9]

These suggestions are useful, but they cannot be allowed to detract from the primary selling goal of the wellness project, which is to offer students better options for nutrition and physical activity. Dealing with specifics such as portion sizes early on may lead to potential supporters dropping out because of too much minutiae.

• In my reading of the Center for Ecoliteracy and NANA policy guides, I found no recommendations for schools to have in place what I call the necessary support systems and health screenings for students with health issues, such as being overweight and obese. Again, I believe good ideas, such as a wellness policy, will not be successful without skilled professionals operating in the trenches, as hectic high school life is described by teachers, to quickly identify students who need intervention, professionals such as the Moorhead High School Wellness

Team of Barbara Grant, Nancy Clifford, Brad Langdon, Tony Jankowski, Marge Edgar, Martha Mayer, and Harry Polk. There need to be doers like Al Morris in the school who don't look the other way when they observe a student like Dylan headed for trouble. Educators can talk all day about the need to provide better nutrition and physical activity for students. I argue that these good ideas will fail unless they are backed up by skilled professionals who are committed to making these needed programs a reality.

- There is no mention in these guides of how schools can deal with the resistance by some staff, students, parents, and school alumni to improving nutrition and physical activity for students, resistance that I believe is sure to come. For example, some members of the teaching staff will object to being asked to serve as personal adult advisors to students and to intervene when they observe a student with health and well-being problems. Some counselors will object to the creation of new counseling roles that focus on quick intervention for students through individual and group counseling. Some physical education teachers will object to the "new" physical education approach that offers vigorous exercise; screening for high blood pressure, blood sugar, and cholesterol; weight reduction intervention; and a regular report card for students identifying their overall physical well-being. Some cafeteria workers will object to having dietitians brought on board, being retrained to prepare healthy foods, and being required to learn about adolescent development and how to interact with teens in a positive way. Many high school departments have guarded their turf during many budget battles. They have created an "all for one, one for all, we are all in this together" mantra for their staff. Changing that historical pattern and bringing new programs and personnel into advisory, counseling, and physical education roles will require great tact, salesmanship, being clear on "what's in it for me," political will and risk, and steady, inviting perseverance. Let's not forget resistance on the part of students, parents, and alumni. Some students will object to the new nutrition and physical activity programs in the school and say that their nutrition and physical activity are up to them and none of the school's business. Some parents and alumni will object to the effort by the school to limit access to fast food served in nearby restaurants. They will say that eating fast food at local restaurants is a school tradition and a way of life. Again, I believe that the good ideas in the Center for Ecoliteracy and NANA wellness policy guides will never reach the light of day unless school leaders anticipate the reality of such resistance and are ready to tackle it and get resisting staff, students, parents, and community members on board.

• Finally, the NANA recommendations for staff wellness need to be expanded to include institutional support. I believe the recommendations need to move beyond "personal efforts by staff to maintain a healthy lifestyle." Personal responsibility is not enough. Staff, like students, need daily, easily accessible institutional support and incentives such as workshops on healthy nutrition, screening for health risks, vigorous physical activity, health and wellness information, and easily accessible sources of support and help in the school and community.

I believe these suggestions can add some clarity to how best to sell and deliver education reforms such as local wellness policies. I would also caution educators to keep in mind that the process of implementing the good ideas about how to improve the nutrition and physical activity of students will not happen overnight and without heavy resistance and battles. The fight for wellness at the national level will be led by powerful lobbying groups who will raise vigorous challenges to serving students healthier foods.

One example is the Center for Consumer Freedom, a nonprofit advocacy group financed by the food and restaurant industry, who charge that their clients are being unfairly blamed for making Americans fat and unhealthy.[10] Rick Berman, a Washington lobbyist who runs the center, says that people are smart enough to make their own well-informed choices.[11] The food industry has an annual revenue of $550 billion and derives huge profits from products most nutritionists frown on.[12] The National Restaurant Association's president, Steven Anderson, said in June 2005, "Food establishments should not be blamed for issues of personal responsibility and freedom of choice."[13] Writer Derrick Z. Jackson suggests this rhetoric of "choice" is meant to obscure obesity's 112,000 deaths a year.[14]

These are expected attacks. But as I have suggested in this chapter, implementation of local wellness policies will not happen without many turf battles. Students, parents, teachers, and even administrators don't like change, and those who are the messengers for change are easy targets. If creating local wellness policies evolves as other education reforms do, the leaders in this kind of effort will no doubt experience professional and personal attacks from resisting critics. The *Boston Globe* reports that the amount of time allotted for lunch in Massachusetts high schools went from 31.8 minutes in 2003 to 26.7 minutes in 2005. The primary reason for the lunchtime reduction was making more time in the schedule for academics.[15] Efforts to reverse this trend, and similar challenges, will not be easy. Reform is not fun and games and is not for the faint of heart. One can offer suggestions from afar for such a process, but only those in the school understand how intense the heat of the battle can get.

The American Heart Association can state "we need to take action" and "attacking the obesity problem means focusing extra attention upon those at greatest risk."[16] But implementing policies and plans to take action can become very nasty when change is in the offing and it involves your turf. I believe the key to success is convincing educators on the front lines that their intervention offers our best chance to succeed in this call for action and that schools do indeed need to make sure the daily schedule offers students the opportunity for healthy nutrition and vigorous physical activity as well as academic challenges. Both health and academic learning opportunities are necessary to developing competent and healthy future citizens. Time and support must be found for each. In the end, caring, alert, and skilled educators represent our best opportunity to help prevent illness, not merely treat it after the fact. Risa Lavizzo-Mourey, president and CEO of the Robert Wood Johnson Foundation, suggests, "When it comes to obesity we truly face a public health threat of epidemic proportions. We need to change course so we don't raise the first generation of American kids who will live sicker and die younger than the generations before them."[17]

REDESIGNING THE SCHOOL CAFETERIA SO IT BECOMES A SETTING WHERE STUDENTS WANT TO BE IS A CRITICAL FIRST STEP FOR ADMINISTRATORS AND WELLNESS LEADERS

Reporter Ben Feller suggests that educators throughout America are testifying to the worth of friendly school design. In schools style is taking on substance. From the width of corridors to the depth of classroom sinks, the smallest detail is viewed as a way to foster an academic advantage. At Manassas Park High School, scores in algebra, geometry, and writing have risen since 1999 when students moved into a building featuring light, versatility, and open spaces. High school principal Bruce McDade, who is in charge of student learning, morale, and safety, says he has no doubt the physical features have contributed to these scores. "That's exactly the message," McDade said. "The design of this building does in fact have a measurable effect on student achievement and student behavior."[18]

Feller states that studies support what educators consider to be common sense: "Students do better in schools where they hear well, see well and are not packed into tight spaces. Noise, light, air quality, cold and heat have all been found to influence behavior." Feller suggests that the conversation about school construction is changing and school leaders are asking new questions, such as "What kind of layout would students find so engaging it would make them eager to show up?" and "What do parents and teachers want?" and "How can the community help design a new setting?" Ronald Bogle, president of the American Architectural Foundation and former president of the Oklahoma Board of Education, urges school districts to "create environments that are uplifting, that are exciting, that are interesting."[19]

In proceeding to redesign the school cafeteria so it becomes an attractive setting and a desired destination for students, I urge the school wellness team to keep the following comments in mind:

- Listen to groups of students, staff, parents, and community members concerning what kind of layout students would find so engaging that it would make them eager to show up. Betty Bender, food service director in Dayton, Ohio, public schools and winner of the 2005 Gold Plate Award for Food Service Operator of the Year, given annually by the International Food Service Manufacturers' Association, suggests that this kind of assessment is important in that it helps to "know your customers and involve them in your program."[20] Reporter Ralph E. Vincent applauds efforts of food service personnel to know their customers because with the growth of the fast-food industry, school food service managers have found themselves in stiff competition with slick advertising, fancy food displays, and split-second service.[21] Even in schools where kids cannot leave school grounds for the restaurant down the street, the impact of the fast-food revolution is felt. Bender advises, "Keep an eye on the competition."[22]
- Ready students for the opportunity to get involved early on in the menu planning through taste and advisory panels. Shirley Watkins, director of food and nutrition services for the Memphis, Tennessee, city schools, says that in the spring of 2005 a student advisory group tasted test foods to determine what items the food service staff would buy for the first half of the upcoming school year. In the past, Watkins suggests, "We were not astute enough to find healthy substitute items for them or ask them before we planned the menu what they'd like to have. Keeping tuned in to what kids want is not only helpful, it's essential."[23]
- Be aware that the physical environment of the cafeteria and the tone set by staff may be more important to students than the food served. Betty Bender says that part of what their fast-food competitors are offering children is a noninstitutional place to eat.[24] While school food service directors don't usually

have the freedom and resources to make dining areas what they would like them to be, making a few changes can make a big difference in students' attitudes. A survey of one of the high schools in Memphis showed just how important the serving environment is.[25] Bender says, "The students' greatest complaints were the decorations in the cafeteria, the noise and the lack of supervision. We had more comments about appearances than we did about food. I was surprised."[26] Charles Tutt, school food director for Colorado Springs, Colorado, knows that some improvements have paid off in increased student participation in the school lunch program. He says, "We have an advisory committee here and we asked them to go out and convince the principals that they had to give kids more time to eat and that the kids needed a nice, comfortable environment. They've done this and our participation is up eight to ten percent."[27] Still, Tutt reminds members of wellness teams that in the effort to provide healthy food to students in an attractive environment, they need to offer concrete ways to bring outdated cafeteria rooms, furniture, and facilities up to date so they can attract students. He says,

I have a high school smack downtown with a kitchen and dining room on the fourth floor. There's a beautiful view of the mountains, but the building was built sixty years ago and has not been touched in sixty years, paint or anything. The furniture is at least thirty years old. It's a dungeon up there and I can't get 150 kids to eat lunch there. All the fast food restaurants are across the street and the kids are going out. We've got kids in that building who have never been up to the cafeteria, and I don't blame them. It's one of our better cafeteria operations but I don't want to eat there.[28]

• There are secondary school food service models that are successful even though they have spaces that are problematic. Tutt says that in one high school, "The cafeteria room is absolutely atrocious. It's two-and-a-half stories high and looks like a gymnasium with lots of metal. But they've sectioned off the rooms down on the lower level and made it a very warm, comfortable area with walnut-grain tables and orange chairs." Tutt also describes a junior high cafeteria that has "a regular one-story room with a stage in it. All along one wall there are windows that look out at Pike's Peak. The interior walls are brick and the tables are walnut with bright golden-rod-colored chairs. It's also a very warm, comfortable dining room."[29]

- Some cafeteria improvements can be made easily. Betty Bender, Shirley Watkins, and Charles Tutt suggest changes like painting murals on the wall, purchasing chairs that have warm, fall-type colors such as orange, and having attractive serving displays that add color and warmth to the cafeteria.[30] Shirley Watkins also suggests,

> It is important for school service people to try to make the serving area appealing. The way the food is merchandised and positioned in the steam tables can help remove the institutional atmosphere. Merchandising doesn't cost a lot of money. You can use things you already have, such as fresh vegetables and fresh fruits for garnishes. You can perk up any food and make it appetizing and appealing.[31]

- A review of the offerings of professional food service organizations can also help local wellness teams generate new ideas for their cafeteria. Aramark School Support Services has designed a U.B.U. lounge concept to get teens excited about lunch. According to reporter Joan Lang, Aramark's research found that 93% of high school students said they wanted to spend time with their friends at lunch. To that end, Aramark developed the U.B.U. lounge concept for high school cafeterias. U.B.U. is open all day and has an area designed to look like a modern living room with couches for chilling out with friends. Serving and dining areas sport bright neon decor and graphic elements and an "Expression Wall" that touts being yourself. Lively music and casual staff uniforms complete the image that "everyone fits in," even employees.[32]

- As Betty Bender suggests, the helpfulness of food service personnel is key in revitalizing the school cafeteria.[33] Her advice should be a major part of the wellness team effort. However, as Marilyn Briggs, a nationally recognized leader in food service and nutrition research, writes,

> Food service is often the last district partner to be brought into the change process, but it is the one upon which all others rely for success. School districts should plan on implementing a program of professional development for food service staff. Professional development is a direct and critical investment in the individuals the district is counting on to make the change.

For example, Briggs suggests,

> New menus may require food service employees to learn new skills. The menus the district tends to serve will tell you what skill the food service staff need to acquire. It is also true that food service employees' jobs become more rewarding and satisfying when the work is less routine and requires skillful execution. It is through professional development that food service staff acquires those valuable and transferable skills that might qualify for higher pay. When food service staff find the work more satisfying and receive the respect they deserve, enthusiasm will build for the new program. At the policy level, I would advocate for better pay for food service staff, and development of some professional requirements and expectations for anyone who is involved in the preparation of food for children. These would include cooking skills, basic sanitation and safety training.[34]

In the end a commonsense approach appears to be the best plan for a school's wellness team. Reporter Vincent sums up this approach by suggesting what is needed to increase student participation: good food, nice surroundings, nice people. He says, "What kids want at school is not that different from most of us want when we're eating away from home."[35] Shirley Watkins adds another critical component. She says, "We want to make sure lunchtime is a happy time. It's the one time children get a chance to really enjoy themselves during the day, because school really isn't always a lot of fun for children. When they get to the cafeteria, it should be a place that has a good atmosphere and it should be fun."[36]

However, Marilyn Briggs offers a dose of reality when she states, "The lunch period has more often been regarded as time stolen away from the curriculum, rather than part of the curriculum. We need to make school meals part of a nutritional education program. That connection feels self-evident, but schools and districts have been slow to make it."[37]

MAKE IT EASY TO IMPLEMENT HEALTHY EATING AND DRINKING INITIATIVES FOR STUDENTS BY CONSIDERING A WHOLE SCHOOL FOOD SERVICE MODEL THAT OFFERS A WIDE VARIETY OF EATING CHOICES THROUGHOUT THE SCHOOL DAY

I believe school wellness teams can learn a great deal about revitalizing school food service from research gathered in the United Kingdom. The Food in Schools program's Whole School approach to healthy eating was developed in the United Kingdom to offer support to schools in tackling childhood obesity. The program is a joint venture between the Department of Health (DH) and the Department of Education and Skills (DES) to help make healthier food choices an integral part of the school day. This initiative was prompted by concerns over the current and future health and well-being of school children, particularly the rising levels of obesity and diet-related conditions.

The Whole School approach is based on the notion that because children spend a quarter of their waking day in school, one big step to improving the nutrition of children is to offer and promote healthy food and drink choices throughout the school day. The school environment, attitudes of staff and pupils, and what children learn in the classroom have a major influence on their knowledge and understanding of health. If encouraged to enjoy healthy food and drink early on, it is much more likely that these positive behaviors will remain with a child throughout life. *Food in Schools: The Essential Guide* advises that one of the most important considerations for implementing healthy eating and drinking initiatives in school is to make it easy. The guide states, "There is no simple solution and 'one' size doesn't fit all."[38]

With this in mind, the Department of Health ran eight pilot programs in over three hundred primary, middle, secondary, and special education schools to determine key features to establishing successful and sustainable healthy eating initiatives in schools. The pilots included Healthier Breakfast Clubs, Tuck Shops, Water Provision, Vending Machines, the Dining Room Environment, Cookery Clubs, and Growing Clubs. A Healthier Breakfast Club provides an opportunity for pupils and staff to eat breakfast together in a stimulating environment; has a positive effect on pupil concentration and performance throughout the day; engages pupils in making healthier choices about diet by providing them with encouragement, knowledge, and support; can help improve pupil attendance and punctuality; can lead to better social interactions and skills between pupils; increases the contact between teachers and parents; can improve pupils' motivation and self confidence through relationships with teachers; and can benefit low-income families by providing no-cost or low-cost breakfast.[39]

A case study in the Food in Schools data describes how a breakfast club was launched in a secondary school in a deprived area with high unemployment to kick-start a whole-school approach to healthier eating. A drop-in café was opened, called "Switch on to Breakfast," where pupils could eat breakfast, listen to music, and watch TV. The informal environment was liked by pupils and made the club feel less like school. In the United Kingdom, 12% to 17% of teens have nothing to eat before school. "It's sociable to be sitting down and talking while eating. It gives us somewhere to go," is a recurring theme in Food in Schools feedback data from students. Another case study in the Food in Schools report describes a breakfast club that was set up in a special school. Pupils were responsible for setting up the club, naming it the "Chill Out Zone." The kitchen supervisor helps pupils prepare and serve meals. She also trains pupils in food hygiene.[40]

Healthier Breakfast Clubs appear to provide an excellent model because they provide pupils with somewhere to go, a place to socialize with peers and staff, and easy access to healthy food and drink. While "one size doesn't fit all," a key factor in the success of breakfast clubs appears to be promoting the social aspects for pupils and keeping it simple, in a real sense providing pupils with a home away from home in an atmosphere that is calm and happy, a place where they can come on a regular basis, where they can be be valued and known by peers and staff, and where they feel they belong and are part of a community that cares for everyone's well-being.

The Food in Schools report also suggests that Healthier Breakfast Clubs could also include an area where pupils can listen to music, play computer and board games, use computers to do research and homework projects, join with peers to share hobbies, and read newspapers, books, and magazines on health and adolescent life.[41] In my readings about breakfast clubs, the image that comes to mind is a dining area in a home that exudes love and care for family members by creating conditions for all members to be noticed, affirmed, and listened to, and to enjoy healthy food and drink that prepares them for the day ahead, knowing that while there may be difficulties that arise, they can return to this place to renew their strength and hope. It is an image that is not familiar to many students, like Dylan. I am not suggesting that schools become another home for teenagers. However, schools can create many of the positive conditions found in a loving and caring home, conditions that can contribute to the improvement of a student's health and well-being as well as academic achievement.

These are the critical elements school wellness leaders need to include in their plan to attract and sustain student involvement. I believe that while school cafeterias need to serve a nutritional menu that includes cereal, fruit, vegetables, breads, skim milk and dairy foods, healthy drinks, and so forth, the key to success appears to be also creating a setting with a welcoming menu, a noninstitutional setting where students want to be, where they can socialize, and where they can get a healthy respite to ready themselves for the academic and personal challenges that await them at school and at home.

The Food in Schools guide suggests creating Tuck Shops in schools as an important component in the Whole School approach. Tuck Shops provide an opportunity for pupils to purchase a range of food and drink that provides a source of energy and refreshment during their break time. A healthier Tuck Shop should reflect healthier eating and drinking messages by offering a wide range of foods that will be able to complement other foods eaten throughout the school day at breakfast and lunch. As the report suggests, no single food can provide all the necessary ingredients. Variety is important. Break-time sales might include drinks such as water, skim milk, fruit drinks, and yogurt drinks. Fruits and vegetables might include bananas, pears, carrot sticks, and clementines. Specials for the day might include dried fruit bars, fruit and cheese scones, sandwiches and baguettes, yogurt, low-sugar cereal bars, and currant buns. Tuck Shops usually operate out of the dining area. In many cases the Tuck Shop may simply be a table or trolley placed in a convenient location. The venue of the Tuck Shop should be warm and welcoming, using brightly colored plastic tablecloths, displaying items in wicker baskets or colored bowls, having music playing in the background, and displaying interesting and informative posters.[42]

The pilot projects also demonstrated that pupils' consumption of water during the school day can be increased. According to the Food in Schools guide, data from the Water Provision pilot programs suggest there is strong evidence that the project was successful in increasing levels of water consumption. In the water provision pilot, 82% of primary and 65% of secondary schools reported increased consumption. Preference for drinking water over other drinks rose 1.6 times in primary schools and 1.4 times in secondary schools, where preference for carbonated soft drinks fell. Teachers also reported that the enhanced water provision contributed to a more settled and productive learning environment, as well as helping to instill good habits. The pilot project's data suggest that water can provide a plentiful source of low-cost refreshment throughout the school day; reduce tiredness, irritability, and distraction from thirst; have a positive effect on pupil concentration throughout the day; and raise awareness of the importance of adequate fluid intake and healthy eating as part of a healthy, active lifestyle. Water provision in the school means providing good quality water, providing water free of charge, ensuring that hygienic, modern water sources are available and maintained, and promoting good habits of water consumption during the day. The Food in Schools guide recommends that pupils and staff drink six to eight cups of water during the day. Schools can use different methods, such as bottled water coolers, traditional water fountains, and point-of-use coolers that are part of many schools' main water supply.[43]

How best to utilize vending machines to provide healthy eating and drinking habits for pupils was also a major component in the Whole School pilot projects. The data from the project were extremely positive and suggest vending machines can indeed play a major role in the Whole School approach when they are stocked with healthy food and drink that is attractively packaged. Vending machines help expand existing food provisions offered at breakfast, break time, lunch, and after school; offer a "grab and go" opportunity for busy pupils; reduce long lines at peak lunch periods; help keep pupils on site during the day; may generate income for the school; and signal that vendors from the community are committed to supporting the Whole School approach to healthier food and drink for pupils. The Food in Schools guide advances the commonsense notion that many schools have vending machines and although vending has been criticized in the past, there is no reason why vending machines cannot provide a range of food that is healthier and supports the Whole School approach. The guide advocates that vending should not be looked at in isolation but as part of the planning in the Whole School service. The vending machines should reflect the objectives of the Whole School policy and offer such items as fresh fruit, dried fruits, fruit salads, filled rolls, sandwiches and baguettes, salads, pasta mixes, breakfast cereal, skim milk, yogurt, pizza slices with less cheese, water, fruit juices, and yogurt drinks.[44]

How schools can improve the lunchtime dining experience was also a major component in the Whole School approach. The Dining Room Environment pilot project demonstrated that changes in the dining environment can have an immediate, significant, and sustainable impact on healthy eating. The data from the pilot project describe an inner-city school where the dining room had been changed into a burger bar five years ago. This resulted in low uptake of school meals, especially the healthier options, and greater truancy after lunch. As part of the pilot project, the dining room was redecorated with its bright colors toned down. A variety of health posters and information was displayed around the room and new menu boards were put up. The dining area began serving a range of healthy sandwiches and more traditional meals. Pupils were receptive to the changes and to the healthier eating initiatives.[45]

The Food in Schools guide suggests that schools have found focusing on their dining room to be invaluable in terms of changing culture, ethos, and understanding of healthier eating messages. Research shows that pupils' surroundings have an impact on their sense of well-being. Judicious use of color, images, messages, information, well-planned seating, and music can have an enormous effect on the sense of "space." To develop healthier eating habits, pupils must respect and enjoy the environment they are in as well.[46]

The guide also suggests that pupils, like everyone else, appreciate and are motivated to select their eating environment by a number of strategies employed in the commercial sector, including good customer service, speedy service, multiple pay points, pictorial and descriptive menus, appropriate and plentiful menu options, a pleasant dining environment, perceived value for money, and attractively presented food and drink. By ensuring that pupils eat lunch in a school that has a balanced and varied menu, schools are more likely to be able to influence the type of food and drinks consumed, thereby improving health. A successful dining room makeover is all about good design. The logistics of waiting in line, serving, paying, eating, and clearing up should be embedded in the design from the outset. No amount of cheerful displays will tempt pupils if they are frustrated by having to sacrifice too much of their lunch time waiting in line.[47] And I would add that no healthy and attractive menu items will tempt students either if they spend much of their precious lunch time waiting in line.

If educators are going to motivate students to try healthier food and drinks, they need to provide a setting that students respect and enjoy. That is the only way students will become stakeholders in revitalizing the school cafeteria and food service. It is no surprise that one of the recommendations of the dining room environment project is to remind schools that "if pupils are allowed out over the lunch time period, external influences pose a challenge. Bakeries, cafes, chip shops and other takeout eating are all in competition with the school dining room. If pupils are not allowed out at lunch time, they might purchase food and drink on the way to school due to problems of long lines and/or the short lunch break."[48]

How to involve pupils as stakeholders in the Whole School approach is also highlighted in the project description. The Food in Schools guide reports that Healthier Cookery Club pilot projects provide an opportunity for pupils, staff, families, and the local community to work together to prepare healthy food, eat together, and learn about healthy eating and food hygiene in an enjoyable and dynamic way. A cookery club offers the opportunity for participants to learn practical food skills. This often builds on what pupils learn in the formal curriculum. Through the cookery club it is hoped that pupils will enjoy cooking, enjoy eating what food they make, learn basic food skills, apply food hygiene and healthy eating messages, and embrace other cultures.[49]

Cookery clubs also provide excellent opportunities to practice and apply basic skills such as communication, literacy, and numeracy as well as practical problem-solving skills. Messages from cookery clubs can also help parents and members of the family see the potential of a healthier diet. If pupils take home food they have cooked in the club and share it with their families, this may give parents the confidence to offer their children a more varied diet. Cookery clubs often run after school on a weekly basis or on weekends and use the school dining area. Some schools combine sports with healthier eating by preparing food in the cookery clubs that is served after the sporting event is over. A case study in the Food in Schools guide describes a cookery club that was set up

following the results of a questionnaire sent out to pupils and parents to assess knowledge of healthier eating, food hygiene and safety. The club recipes were based on fruit and vegetables and tasting sessions were run for participants to try food they were not familiar with. The cookery club took place in a local secondary school's food technology classroom. The use of the secondary school's facilities was felt to have contributed to the success of the club.[50]

The pilot project's evaluations found that creating a fun and social environment successfully engaged students in selecting, preparing, and trying healthier foods. In addition, the clubs improved social and interpersonal skills of pupils through teamwork, the responsibility of running a club, and a feeling of achievement from creating a dish from start to finish.[51]

Using Growing Clubs also proved to be a successful way to involve pupils as stakeholders in the Whole School approach. The Food in Schools guide states that a Growing Club gives pupils the opportunity to plan, sow, tend, and harvest a range of fruits and vegetables at school. It extends pupils' understanding of food chain issues by bringing the process directly under their control. Whether the club is run as part of the formal school curriculum or as an extracurricular activity, it should be seen as a vital teaching and learning experience for pupils.[52]

The Growing Club also makes use of the school grounds, which are additional learning spaces at school. It provides an area of interest for the entire school community and can be shown to guests and visitors as a key feature of the school. It also provides an ideal vehicle to promote healthier eating and drinking messages to pupils. In time, the Growing Club can also produce a number of crops that can be eaten in school, perhaps in the Tuck Shop or Cookery Club. The guide suggests that schools do not need a large garden area to cultivate the favorite foods of pupils and staff. A well-planned growing club can use containers, grow-bags, and hanging baskets. Growing Clubs in schools is a part of the UK government–sponsored Growing Schools program, a program that aims to harness the full potential of the outdoor classroom as a teaching and learning resource. The program focuses in particular on food, farming, and ensuring that pupils are given first-hand experience in the natural world around them and that outdoor learning activities are integrated into everyday teaching practice.[53]

All the components in the Whole School approach may not be doable in every secondary school in the United States. As the Food in Schools guide suggests, no one size fits all. Some schools will face barriers such as limited financing, outdated facilities, inadequate staffing, and so forth, while others are ready to embrace the Whole School approach. Students in schools that follow the lead of the Whole School model will be fortunate. They will be part of a daily experience that offers them many options to eat and learn about healthy food and drink in a dining area that they respect and enjoy. And they will be able to gather concrete experiences in making and growing food through activities such as cookery and growing clubs. In the process they will have the ongoing opportunity to share these experiences with peers and adults in the school—teachers, administrators, and support staff—and become part of a school community in which the health and well-being of each member is valued. When students such as Dylan are observed heading toward the margins of school life and developing health problems such as obesity, help is on the way. While this is not the case in many schools today, school wellness teams need to press on and give their best effort to creating even a small piece of the Whole School program. The ideas in the Food in Schools guide are doable, and they appear to be successful approaches to help address in a concrete, ongoing way student obesity and related health problems that negatively impact on academic achievement and personal development.

There are students like Dylan in every high school in America. We need to find ways to give them the same lifeline provided by Al Morris and the Moorhead High Wellness Team. Picture for a moment what this can mean for Dylan and his peers.

Dylan arrives early to school. He heads toward the Breakfast Club, where he is welcomed by newly made friends he met at the after-school Cookery Club, run by dietitian Nancy Clifford. The Cookery Club also meets on Saturday mornings. Parents are invited to the Saturday sessions. Margo has been able to participate on two occasions and has begun using some of the menus at home. On this particular morning there is a birthday celebration for Roberto Diaz, who is turning fourteen. Student volunteers from the birthday club have made a carrot cake, and there are yogurt, fruit drinks, cereal, skim milk, breads, and hot drinks available. Nurse Barbara Grant and counselor Brad Langdon are on hand for the festivities. Dylan knows he will get the same kind of treatment when his birthday comes up in December.

In homeroom he talks with advisor Martha Mayer about how things are going at school and at home. Martha makes it a point to give Dylan some special time about once a week. Later in the morning Dylan has a fourth-period break and heads to the dining area for a Café Break. Al Morris and the Wellness Team thought using the term "Tuck Shop" might not fit at Moorhead High, but they are using the same concept of providing a healthy break to energize students. Dylan is using the short break between periods to reach his goal of drinking six to eight bottles of water during the school day.

At lunchtime Dylan resists the pressure from some of his old friends to go out to a local fast-food restaurant. He has learned how to handle these kinds of pressures in his individual and group counseling sessions with Brad Langdon. But it still takes great effort on his part to say, "No, I am eating in the dining area. It's better for my weight program." He has tried to encourage some of his old friends to eat in school but with little success. Brad Langdon keeps telling him to focus on what *he* needs. Maybe his old friends will follow his lead later on. At lunch Dylan eats a fresh vegetable salad made from the Growing Club's and Farm-to-School Program's farm produce, a tuna sandwich with low-fat mayonnaise, and a fresh fruit salad, accompanied by fruit juice and water again. After school he stops by a vending machine for more fruit juice and an apple on his way to a workout class led by physical education teachers Tony Jankowski and Marge Edgar. The workout period includes having Nurse Grant and an intern from Moorhead Hospital regularly monitor his blood pressure, blood sugar, and cholesterol level.

On the way to the gym, Al Morris reminds Dylan to tell his mother about the parent support group meeting that evening at 8:00 and that he wants Dylan to serve on a welcoming committee for new students. Dylan has become very involved at Moorhead High. He also attends a once-a-week tutorial on healthy eating and diet led by Nancy Clifford and is a member of the 48-Hour Program, led by Barbara Grant, that offers support during the weekend to maintain a healthy diet, refrain from tobacco and alcohol, and learn how to seek peers and activities that promote a healthy lifestyle. Dylan's sister Kate and brother Kyle are also involved in support programs in the junior high and, like Dylan, can't wait to get to their Breakfast Club every morning. They are all chipping in to make healthy dinner meals to take the load off Margo, who is taking courses for a diploma in the evening and attending the weekly parent support group.

Is this pie-in-the-sky thinking? A fantasy? Hardly. The whole-school-day interventions that are available to Dylan are doable. They are not just *good ideas* to be placed on the shelf but rather concrete ways to offer an open door to teens who educators sense are heading toward unhealthy lifestyles, dropping out, and the possibility of an early death. In my experience in the schools, I have witnessed similar turnarounds by students such as Dylan, Kate, and Kyle and parents like Margo, who were slowly slipping into poor health and despair. The key to successful interventions to address teen obesity and related health and personal problems is creating the same conditions that are present in a loving and caring home—a place where kids are known well; are valued for their differences; are given many opportunities to share their daily life stories, both good and bad; can enjoy healthy food and drink in an environment they respect and in which they feel wanted; and can contribute as a team member by sharing in the healthy menu planning, cooking, and clearing up; and where problems are solved around the dining room table, not avoided or softened by the use of tobacco, alcohol, or drugs.

According to nutrition and health expert Dr. Karen Weber Cullen, researchers at the University of Minnesota reported that teens who ate seven or more meals with their families each week generally had higher grade point averages and were less likely to feel depressed, drink alcohol, smoke cigarettes, or use marijuana than those who ate less than twice a week with their families.[54] I believe programs such as the Whole School approach can have the same health benefits for students, in that the eating and drinking experience is shared with caring adults and peers in an attractive, happy environment that they respect. Available and caring educators and peers can create conditions in schools that are similar to the family dining room table. Isn't this the kind of school dining experience many readers wanted for themselves as teenagers? Today's teens are no different.

THERE ARE EDUCATORS AND SCHOOLS BREAKING NEW GROUND TO OFFER STUDENTS BETTER NUTRITION IN CREATIVE WAYS

Reporter Kim Severson describes the efforts by educators at Promise Academy, a charter school in Harlem, New York City, where "food is as important as homework." In 2004 school officials took control of students' diets, dictating a regimen of unprocessed, regionally grown food at school and, as much as possible, at home. Almost 90% of students at the school come from families poor enough to qualify for free government lunches and 44% are overweight.[55]

Geoffrey Canada, the teacher and author who developed the Promise Academy, says, "Our challenge is to create an environment where young people actually eat healthy and learn to do it for the rest of their lives." Promise Academy is part of a sixty-block "Children's Zone," a tight web of social, health, and educational programs in Harlem. The school has longer hours than most public schools and runs through much of the summer. School officials regularly monitor the students' weight and fitness along with their academic progress. In terms of school meals, the goal is to serve two meals and two snacks a day to the 1,300 students who will eventually fill the school. The wellness team at the school uses strict guidelines, education, and a little psychology to change young palates. One key is to teach resistance to marketing come-ons from fast-food companies and candy manufacturers.[56]

According to Severson, eating at the Promise Academy is about more than just food. Students learn to respect where it comes from and who serves it, as well as whom they eat with. They must use tongs to pick up their morning bagel. They may not bang their trays down on the cloth-covered cafeteria tables. No one is allowed to toss whole peaches or cut in line. The kitchen at the academy does not use foods like processed cheese or peanut butter, choosing instead to spend part of the budget in favor of fresher food. The kitchen feeds the students breakfast, lunch, and an array of after-school and Saturday snacks at a daily cost of $5.87 per student. However, even at the Promise Academy, getting students to embrace healthy eating has been a struggle. At first they went home complaining that they had not had enough to eat or that the food was terrible. Andrew Benson, the chef at the school, responded by bringing parents in for a meal. The intervention by Benson helped to quiet student and parent resistance. As parent Jacqueline Warner reported, "It's just that my son wasn't used to eating healthy portions."[57] Severson reports that Ms. Warner has diabetes. She grew up in Harlem, eating what her mother could afford and knew how to cook. Often that meant fried foods, macaroni and cheese, and lots of rice and potatoes. She loved it but attributes her disease, in part, to that diet. She says, "I'm just glad he has a chance to know the difference between food we grew up on and the healthy kind of food they serve in that school."[58]

Epiphany School in Dorchester, Massachusetts, presents another example of a school that incorporates some components of the Whole School approach. Education writer Megan Tench reports that Epiphany, with eighty fifth-to-eighth graders, runs nearly twelve hours a day, eleven months a year. The school's head and cofounder John Finley IV says, "The goal is to be everything a family needs."[59] Epiphany is located in an area of Dorchester that has a high poverty rate and where children often find chaos, neglect, and violence. It is also an area that is devoid of role models and even warm meals and housing. Tench reports that the school has tried to create a competing and almost all-encompassing universe where students cannot only learn but also grow up. For example, on weekdays the students spend from 7:30 a.m. to 7:15 p.m. at the school. After classes end at 3:15 p.m., students play sports until dinner at 5:00 p.m. From 5:30 to 7:15, or until their parents pick them up, they do their homework. Healthy meals are served at breakfast, lunch, and dinner; at dinnertime they use real silverware and plates instead of lunch trays. Parents and siblings are encouraged to dine alongside the students. The school also provides comprehensive health care for students. Once enrolled, students are screened for vision and dental problems and have access to community counseling and mental health services. The school is also open on Saturday, providing students with cooking and dance classes and sports. Field trips are also unique. Every summer Epiphany takes groups of students on extended sailing trips, teaching them about how to work together.[60]

According to Tench, Epiphany has two ironclad requirements. The student's family must be poor enough to qualify for free or reduced-price lunch and, to get parents involved, they must volunteer at least two hours a week at the school on tasks such as preparing meals. One student, fifteen-year-old Josh Simmons, said that getting used to Epiphany's rules and extra-long school day took some time. But the eighth-grader said he feels a special bond with some of the teachers, particularly the nine intern teachers. Josh says, "The interns are kind of close to our age so we can talk to them more than we do an older teacher."[61] In an interview with Tench, Harry Spence, commissioner of the State Department of Social Services, praised the Epiphany program: "It has built powerful relationships between the adults at the school and many of our children, and that's a critical issue because our children have experienced a betrayal or failure of parents to bond with them. So for a school to do that consistently and deeply, it is just a very remarkable thing."[62]

Evidence from both the Promise Academy and the Epiphany School clearly points out that providing students with healthy food and drink in an attractive, safe setting that they respect, where they are known and valued, and where they have the opportunity to form powerful personal relationships with caring and available adults can go a long way toward improving their health and well-being. Clearly,

Promise Academy and Epiphany School are special schools that have emerged to address the health and well-being problems of children in high-poverty areas. They represent the vision of experienced innovators such as Geoffrey Canada, an author and education reformer, and John Finley IV, a Harvard graduate and community activist. They are leaders who have a vision for change, understand how to gather community support to improve the education, health, and well-being of students and can clearly communicate the important idea that student achievement and the opportunity to eat healthy food and drink each day are intertwined.

However, I believe school wellness team members need to keep in mind that efforts to reform the dining experience for students do not require education reformers with proven track records such as Geoffrey Canada and John Finley IV. Nor do approaches to plant the seed for a whole-school approach succeed only in schools that have funding because they have a high percentage of students from poverty areas. Concerned educators in lower-, middle-, and upper-class-area schools can also tap into the growing national feeling that ways have to be found in local schools to improve students' diet and the dining experience in schools. These can be educators who are willing to risk thinking "outside the lunchbox," have a vision for change, and have the political skills needed to gather the support of administrators, colleagues, students, parents, and community members to join in the reform efforts.

Ginny Reale, a health and physical education teacher at East Hampton Middle School in East Hampton, New York, provides such an example. Geraldine Pluenneke reports that a school viewing of the documentary *Super Size Me*, about a man getting heavy and unhealthy after a month of eating fast food, sparked a boycott of the cafeteria fare at East Hampton Middle School.[63] Thirteen-year-old Cailyn Bierley and other students demanded green salads, veggies, and fruit instead of "unhealthy" and "gross" choices like cheeseburgers, pizza, and sugary drinks. They advised students to brown-bag it until the menu improved. Students and staff indicated that up to half the students were participating in the boycott, which began soon after the film was shown. *Super Size Me* was shown to 150 students and their parents in December 2004 as part of a wellness program developed by Ms. Reale to teach students how to eat well, exercise, and avoid smoking. In the film Morgan Spurlock traveled throughout the country discussing the detrimental effects of fast food while on a month-long fast-food-entrée diet. Soon he began to gain weight and experience health problems. In her column, Pluenneke said the boycott might be spreading: "Last week the students in the sixth grade passed out a letter reading, 'Boycott the school lunch. Bring a bagged lunch from home and don't buy anything at the cafeteria.'" School officials said items like cookies and ice cream were to be taken off the menu in September 2005.[64]

Reale told reporter Peter Beller that the boycott began when, the day after the film was shown, some seventh graders linked the film's message about calorie-laden processed food with the menu in the lunchroom and decided to stop buying meals at school.[65] Ms. Reale mentioned the idea to her other classes and the word spread throughout the school, which has an enrollment of 465. Twelve-year-old Devon McGorisk, one of the students who began the boycott, said, "We wrote down a list of foods we wanted." Ms. Reale said the list included more salads, freshly prepared sandwiches, fruit salads, even sushi.[66] Beller indicates in comparison that the menu one day in March 2005 included mozzarella sticks, chicken nuggets, Philly cheese steak sandwiches, ham and cheese melts, muffins, ice cream, small apples, and a fruit cup with three slices of canned peaches. Hamburgers and French fries were sometimes on the menu. Soft drinks were not available, but sugary drinks were. Although students did little to organize a formal protest, lines in the lunchroom started to shrink as word spread.[67]

Although Ms. Reale worried that her students might be taking the healthy eating message too far with a boycott, Gail Parker, the school's principal, insisted on showing the film to the entire school, along with staff members and parents, just before winter break. Parker said, "The cafeteria is saying they have healthy foods available, which is true. But they also have unhealthy foods. We want to eliminate bad choices."[68] Beller points out that while the cafeteria serves salads, sandwiches, wraps and fruit, students and teachers said the healthiest options usually run out quickly. Because the lunch period is only twenty minutes long, common in most schools throughout New York State, students often shun the long lines for the meals in favor of faster, cheaper snack counters where they can grab saucer-sized cookies, fruit snacks, bagels, and sugary drinks.[69]

But Beller says the students' efforts have started to produce results. An anonymous donor gave the school $6,000 to buy a refrigerated display case, which opened for business on April 3, 2005, stocked with tuna and chicken over salad greens, fruit salad, grilled chicken, containers of grapes, and cut vegetables in dip. Ginny Reale's wellness program continues to gather support from principal Gail Parker, faculty, students, parents, and community members. A grant from the East Hampton Healthcare Foundation encourages exercise, healthy lifestyles, eating well, and monitoring of weight and other health indicators, and offers rewards to students who improve their health and well-being.[70]

Teacher Ginny Reale understands that simply lecturing students about healthy food and drink in most cases doesn't bring about needed changes in the dining room experience. She uses the film *Super Size Me* to vividly demonstrate that a steady diet of fast food can be harmful to a student's health. When students tied the message to eat healthier foods with the cafeteria menu, they became involved with a real learning experience on how to use political action to get the cafeteria to serve healthier food. Was she worried and maybe fearful that her teaching initiatives would draw some political heat for her and her students? As Beller's piece suggests, she was worried that students might be carrying the healthy eating message too far with a boycott of the cafeteria menu.

But she had the support of Gail Parker, who sided with her by showing *Super Size Me* to the whole school community—faculty, students, and parents. And Parker came forward and supported Reale's mission without undermining the cafeteria staff. Parker could have taken the easy way out by suggesting that the menu served in the cafeteria was controlled by Whitson's Food Service and out of her hands. She could have made a decision to quash the boycott by putting pressure on Ginny Reale and the students to go slowly.

These are responses that might have been used by administrators before healthy food and drink became a national, state, and local health movement backed up by the vocal groups of educators, parents, community advocates, and, as seen in East Hampton Middle School, students themselves.

Reale and Parker are in tune with our changing times. But they needed each other to bring about necessary change. Chances are that Reale, even with her risk taking, courage, and interest in making East Hampton Middle School a healthier setting, would not have succeeded without the political cover Gail Parker provided for her. She stood behind Reale and was proactive by arranging for student representatives to meet with Whitson's Food Service personnel to advocate for their position. Parker was also instrumental in setting up a meeting of Whitson's representatives with the district's three principals.[71] Chances are that Parker would not have been able to carry out a platform to help students learn a healthier lifestyle unless Ginny Reale decided to take a good idea and throw herself and her students into a concrete plan and action for change. Action matters.

Contrast this success story spearheaded by a caring and savvy teacher and administrator with conditions in the Hempstead, New York, schools. Karla Schuster and Eden Laiken describe a report from the New York State Department of Education in April 2005 indicating that student attendance was low, suspension rates were high, gang activity was conspicuous, the high school's open campus promoted tardiness and absenteeism, the food service had "dirty" cafeterias that served unsafe food lacking in healthy nutrition, and the food director and staff were poorly trained, disregarded basic sanitation, wasted food, inflated the number of meals served, and were unresponsive to parent demands for improvement.[72]

It's no surprise that the high school's open-campus policy led to increased tardiness and absenteeism and that gang activity was there. There is no competing model for students to eat healthy food and drink in an environment that is attractive and that they respect. Who wants to eat in a dirty cafeteria that serves unsafe food lacking in healthy nutrition, served by untrained and unresponsive staff? I wouldn't. Would you? The students at East Hampton Middle School are fortunate that they have educators like Ginny Reale and Gail Parker, who not only care about them but also act to help improve their lives and long-term health. What they offer to their students is no mystery. But it does take a school wellness team that not only has good ideas but also has the will, skills, and courage to make things happen to improve the lives of students. Clearly there is much work to be done in schools like Hempstead High. We need to keep up our efforts to make sure students there get the same respect as students at East Hampton Middle School and that they are encouraged to verbalize their needs like East Hampton students Cailyn Bierley and Devon McGorisk.

NOTES

1. Malin Lundblad, "Corporate Wellness," *OC Metro*, 14 Apr. 2005, http://www.ocmetro.com/archives.ocmetro_2005/metro041405/health041 405.html (accessed 29 Nov. 2005).

2. Michelle R. Davis, "Some Schools Start 'Dieting' Ahead of U.S. Rules," *Education Week*, 5 Jan. 2005, http://www.edweek.org/ew/articles/2005/01/ 05/16wellnessh24.html (accessed 25 May 2005).

3. Janet Brown, "Leadership, Policy, and Change," The Center for Ecoliteracy, 2005, http://www.ecoliteracy.org/publications/rsl.janet_brown.html (accessed 12 Sept. 2005).

4. The Center for Ecoliteracy, "Model Wellness Policy Guide," 1 Sept. 2005, http://www.ecoliteracy.org (accessed 3 Jan. 2006), 1–17.

5. National Alliance for Nutrition and Activity (NANA), "Model Local School Wellness Policies on Physical Activity and Nutrition," Center for Science in the Public Interest, Mar. 2005, http://www.schoolwellness policies.org (accessed 2 June 2005), 1–26.

6. National Alliance for Nutrition and Activity, "Model Local School Wellness Policies," 7.

7. National Alliance for Nutrition and Activity, "Model Local School Wellness Policies," 15.

8. Brown, "Leadership, Policy, and Change," 2.

9. National Alliance for Nutrition and Activity, "Model Local School Wellness Policies," 9, 11.

10. Melanie Warner, "Striking Back at the Food Police," *New York Times,* 12 June 2005, sec. 3, pp. 1, 9.

11. Warner, "Striking Back at the Food Police," sec. 3, pp. 1, 9.

12. Warner, "Striking Back at the Food Police," sec. 3, pp. 1, 9.

13. Warner, "Striking Back at the Food Police," sec. 3, pp. 1, 9.

14. Derrick Z. Jackson, "Why Obesity Is Winning," boston.com, 19 Aug. 2005, http://www.boston.com/news/globe.editorial_opinion/oped/articles/2005/08/19why_obesity (accessed 19 Aug. 2005).

15. *Boston Globe,* "Average Length of Lunch Period in US Schools," boston.com, 6 Aug. 2005, http://www.boston.com/pews/local/articles/2005/08/06lunch (accessed 6 Aug. 2005).

16. American Heart Association, *A Nation at Risk: Obesity in the United States* (Dallas: American Heart Association, 2005), 1.

17. Risa Lavizzo-Mourey, "Obesity Epidemic Is Endangering Our Kids," Robert Wood Johnson Foundation news release, 2005, http://www.rwjf.org/newsroom/featurDetail.jsp?featureID=746&pageNum=2&type=4 (accessed 30 Aug. 2005).

18. Ben Feller, "Educators Testify to Worth of Friendly School Design," *Washington Times,* 7 Nov. 2005, http://www.washtimes.com.php?StoryID=20051106-112220-6594r (accessed 9 Nov. 2005).

19. Feller, "Educators Testify to Worth."

20. Ralph E. Vincent, "Some Advice From Three School Food Service Stars," *Food and Nutrition,* Oct. 1998, http://www.findarticles.com/p/articles/mi_m1098/is_v15ai_3956564 (accessed 23 Oct. 2005).

21. Vincent, "Some Advice."

22. Vincent, "Some Advice."

23. Vincent, "Some Advice."

24. Vincent, "Some Advice."

25. Vincent, "Some Advice."

26. Vincent, "Some Advice."

27. Vincent, "Some Advice."

28. Vincent, "Some Advice."

29. Vincent, "Some Advice."

30. Vincent, "Some Advice."

31. Vincent, "Some Advice."

32. Joan Lang, "Aramark School Support Services: Using Research and Creativity Lounge Rose to the Challenge of Getting Teens Excited About Lunch," *Nation's Restaurant News,* 9 May 2005, http://www.findarticles.com/p/articles/mi_m3190/is_19_39/ai_n1379099 (accessed 23 Oct. 2005).

33. Vincent, "Some Advice."

34. Marilyn Briggs, *Road Map: Rethinking School Lunch Guide*, (Berkeley, CA: The Center for Ecoliteracy, 2005), 1–11.

35. Vincent, "Some Advice."

36. Vincent, "Some Advice."

37. Briggs, *Road Map*, 9.

38. United Kingdom Department of Health (DH) and Department of Education and Skills (DES), *Food in Schools Toolkit* (London: Food in Schools [www.foodinschools.org], 2005), "Why Healthy Eating," 4.

39. United Kingdom DH and DES, *Food in Schools Toolkit*, "Food in School Pilots," 12.

40. United Kingdom DH and DES, *Food in Schools Toolkit*, "Healthier Breakfast Clubs," 14.

41. United Kingdom DH and DES, *Food in Schools Toolkit*, "Healthier Breakfast Clubs," 4.

42. United Kingdom DH and DES, *Food in Schools Toolkit*, "Healthier Tuck Shops," 9.

43. United Kingdom DH and DES, *Food in Schools Toolkit*, "Water Provision," 5.

44. United Kingdom DH and DES, *Food in Schools Toolkit*, "Healthier Vending," 3.

45. United Kingdom DH and DES, *Food in Schools Toolkit*, "Dining Room Environment," 3.

46. United Kingdom DH and DES, *Food in Schools Toolkit*, "Dining Room Environment," 4.

47. United Kingdom DH and DES, *Food in Schools Toolkit*, "Dining Room Environment," 4.

48. United Kingdom DH and DES, *Food in Schools Toolkit*, "Dining Room Environment," 9.

49. United Kingdom DH and DES, *Food in Schools Toolkit*, "Healthier Cookery Clubs," 5.

50. United Kingdom DH and DES, *Food in Schools Toolkit*, "Healthier Cookery Clubs," 14.

51. United Kingdom DH and DES, *Food in Schools Toolkit*, "Healthier Cookery Clubs," 3.

52. United Kingdom DH and DES, *Food in Schools Toolkit*, "Growing Clubs," 5.

53. United Kingdom DH and DES, *Food in Schools Toolkit*, "Growing Clubs," 5.

54. Laurie Tarkan, "Benefits of the Dinner Table Ritual," *New York Times*, 3 May 2005, F9.

55. Kim Severson, "Eating, Writing and 'Rithmetic: Harlem Pupils Meet Swiss Chard," *New York Times*, 9 Sept. 2005, B5.

56. Severson, "Eating, Writing and 'Rithmetic," B5.

57. Severson, "Eating, Writing and 'Rithmetic," B5.

58. Severson, "Eating, Writing and 'Rithmetic," B5.

59. Megan Tench, "In a Struggling Area, a Refuge for Learning," boston.com, 17 Nov. 2005, http://www.boston.com/news/education/k_12/articles/2005/11/27/in_a_struggling_area, (accessed 27 Nov. 2005).

60. Tench, "In a Struggling Area."

61. Tench, "In a Struggling Area."

62. Tench, "In a Struggling Area."

63. Geraldine Pluenneke, "East Hampton Kids Get Results with Super-size Cafeteria Boycott," *Newsday*, 8 Apr. 2005, A3.

64. Pluenneke, "East Hampton Kids," A3.

65. Peter C. Beller, "Boycott or No, Students Get Results," *New York Times*, 10 Apr. 2005, http://query.nytimes.com/gst/fullpage.html?res=9C01E2DC163EF933A25757C0A9639C8 (accessed 5 May 2005).

66. Beller, "Boycott or No."

67. Beller, "Boycott or No."

68. Beller, "Boycott or No."

69. Beller, "Boycott or No."

70. Beller, "Boycott or No."

71. Beller, "Boycott or No."

72. Karla Schuster and Eden Laiken, "Hempstead Gets Low Marks," *Newsday*, 13 Apr. 2005, A14, A15.

5

HOW SCHOOLS CAN INCREASE PHYSICAL ACTIVITY TO HELP STUDENTS REDUCE WEIGHT

Efforts by school wellness teams to provide healthy food and drink need to be accompanied by a plan to increase physical activity for students and regularly monitor important health indicators such as weight and blood pressure. A team effort is needed, such as the one at Moorhead High that involved primary intervention by physical education teachers Tony Jankowski and Marge Edgar, backed up with support from administrator Al Morris, nurse Barbara Grant, counselor Brad Langdon, dietitian Nancy Clifford, and community health and mental health professionals. Ginny Reale's role at East Hampton Middle School fits such a wellness model. She is a health teacher, physical education teacher, and the school's wellness leader.[1] As such, she is a triple-threat interventionist. In health classes she is able to both teach her students how to maintain a daily regimen of physical activity and regularly monitor health indicators with the school nurse. As head of the school wellness program she is able to use her bully pulpit to advise students, faculty, support staff, administrators, and parents on the hows and whys of developing a healthy lifestyle and provide a resource for referrals to community health and mental health agencies.

The intervention roles of Tony Jankowski, Marge Edgar, and Ginny Reale represent a significant shift from a physical education model that mainly focused on athletic teams, a model in which physical activity in gym class was often limited to "throwing out the ball and letting the kids play," as one PE teacher said to me. "Football in the fall, basketball in the winter, softball and baseball in the spring." Gym classes often began with a short lecture by the teacher about the sport of the day, followed by a game led by the more athletic students, while overweight, obese, and poorly coordinated students sat on the bench or played at the fringe of the activity, not involved, not needed, and labeled as losers. While that physical education model, with coaching as the first priority, still exists in some schools, it is giving way to a teaching model that involves students in learning how to be healthier and live longer, more productive lives.

I can relate personally to the hurts that can happen to overweight teens who are deprived of the physical education intervention of caring and savvy teachers such as Jankowski, Edgar, and Reale. I was overweight as a preadolescent. I grew up in the seacoast town of Hull, Massachusetts. Hull's main employer was Paragon Amusement Park, which was located on Nantasket Beach. The park, along with the beach, catered to thousands of day-trippers from the Boston area in the summer and was a bustling place. However, come fall and winter, many local residents were unemployed or trekked into Boston for low-paying jobs. Hull was not a wealthy suburb coveted by educated and successful professionals. It was a blue-collar town with a great deal of poverty and schools that left much to be desired. In fact, there was no high school in Hull. Come grade nine, students were bused to nearby Hingham High School. Hingham was, and is, a wealthy suburban town inhabited by many college-educated families who valued education and encouraged their children to value academic success and seek a college education.

In a sense, there were two worlds in Hingham High. There were the Hull students, who were often poor academic students, had high absentee and truancy rates, brought brown-bag lunches because they couldn't afford to eat a hot lunch in the cafeteria, and had few hopes and dreams for the future except to enter the armed forces. Meanwhile the majority of students from Hingham were successful students, didn't act out by being truant or fighting, dressed in preppy clothes, and had hopes and dreams for the future, a future that included college, not entry into the armed forces or work, as was the case for many Hull students. Still, the "haves" of Hingham and the "have-nots" of Hull did mesh around the athletic teams at the school. Many Hull students like myself found their place through participation in sports and struck up close relationships with coaches who provided mentoring that encouraged teens like me to have hopes and dreams and even consider the possibility that college was possible. More on that later.

I grew up in a family of four children; I was the oldest. We were poor. My dad worked two jobs and our family was barely able to make ends meet, as my mom said. Our daily diet was similar to that of Promise Academy parent Jacqueline Warner[2]—fried foods such as eggs, fish cakes, chicken, hamburgers, and Spam; macaroni and cheese; lots of potatoes and pasta; hot dogs and beans; canned soup; canned fruits; cereal with sugar; drinks with sugar; ice cream; and so forth. Fresh fruits and vegetables were seldom seen. The bag lunches we took to school were usually cheese, peanut butter and jelly, or even bean sandwiches—foods that would fill us up. My daily diet was not much different from that of my peers. We were poor kids from a poor neighborhood, a neighborhood in which many adults were overweight, abused alcohol and tobacco, and were ill with diabetes, heart conditions, and cancers, particularly the men, many of whom died far too early in life. My mother and father were very bright and caring people, but this was the life they knew. Survival was the name of the game, and food was a part of that survival. We ate what was cheap and available. The dining experience was not one to enjoy or to help improve one's health and energy; it was meant to keep one filled and going, doing.

By seventh grade I was overweight, inactive, and not doing well in school. Our school had no regular gym class. Recess meant every guy and gal for himself or herself, with daily fights and bullying. No adult supervision, no games, no sports equipment. Just another place where the main goal was to survive. It was kind of like a prison yard where the inmates are turned loose with no need for an intervention program or plan. It was a "let them work out their hostilities so we won't have to deal with it" approach. In the schoolyard I was called many of the same labels that other overweight kids, like Dylan, experienced. I can still remember them: "Fibkins is a loser, a slob, fatso, pregnant tub." No faculty member or administrator intervened or seemed to care that I was taking a lot of hits from the school bullies. I knew instinctively that I was on my own, but I didn't know I was headed for serious health problems, following in the path of many men in my neighborhood who abused food and alcohol to quiet the demons that come with working too hard and for too many hours to stay just above the poverty line. They were paying the bills, making ends meet, but with no money left over except for taking a summer day trip to the nearby beach for a treat of fried clams and fries, buying a case of beer and a pack of Camel cigarettes on a Friday night, and falling asleep while listening to a Red Sox game or a Celtics basketball game. They were exhausted from a work week in which there was little or no play time or exercise.

The only kids I heard talk about exercise at school were the so-called rich kids. Many of them rode new bikes, knew how to play sports, and talked of play time and outings with their parents. They brought their lunches in colorful lunchboxes, not bags, lunchboxes that were beautifully arranged with fresh fruit, wrapped sandwiches, and insulated drink containers with milk and juice. I envied them their lifestyle. And I was also angry, like many poor teens today, that these kids had it better than I did. I was eating baked bean sandwiches that soaked through my brown bag by lunchtime and wearing Army clothes left over from World War II, while they were eating chicken salad sandwiches with fresh lettuce and tomato and wearing preppy clothes and shoes. And I was angry that many of those kids were thin, not being exposed to the name-calling that goes with being overweight.

However, I can also relate personally and professionally to how teenagers can be helped when a caring and savvy physical education teacher and coach comes into their lives, takes notice of their lack of fitness and well-being, and intervenes to direct them toward a healthier lifestyle. I was helped by three educators who not only taught me to be healthier but also were career models for me. I now work out ninety minutes each day and follow a low-fat diet. I walk outdoors, bike frequently, and use the elliptical machine and weights at a health club, a pattern that began to evolve when physical education teachers Bill Carmichael and Ervin Fieger and coach Ward Donner entered my life. That story explains why I am a champion of rigorous physical activity in our schools.

Recreation director and coach Bill Carmichael came into my life in ninth grade. Bill was hired to start a recreation program for the youth in town at the new junior high gym. Bill was a veteran who went to college after serving in the Army. He played college football and received a degree in physical education and recreation. But Bill was no ordinary beginning teacher. He was married with three children, very mature, and had a day job at a residential home for teens. He exuded confidence, was a guy who knew his way around the world, and had a welcoming, supportive demeanor. Word quickly got around the town that Bill was offering something special at the gym. In a matter of months the gym was crowded every night from Monday through Friday. As one of my friends said, "Forget the homework; let's go have fun." Clearly the majority of teens at the evening gym, like myself, were not on the road to academic success. Many of us skipped school at Hingham High at least once a week and headed into Boston to spend the day hanging out in movie theaters and even bars. We were using and abusing alcohol and tobacco bought for us by older classmates. School was a place one had to go, but many teens in our neighborhood lacked academic and career goals and role models. Many Hull students dropped out before graduation. The ones who made it to graduation were often urged to join the armed forces by the school's guidance director. It seemed the only Hull teens to make it to college went on because of the support of their athletic abilities.

So the arrival of Bill Carmichael in the lives of Hull teens was sort of a miracle. Bill quickly organized a three-hour nightly regimen. We learned how to run, play basketball and baseball, lift weights, and do gymnastics; competed athletically with other recreation programs; and took regular field trips to swim at a local college and watch college and professional sports. Bill also made an effort to single out each of the gym participants for praise and to encourage them to value education and have hopes and dreams for the future. He made it a point to encourage healthy eating and drinking and to avoid alcohol and tobacco. Part of that ritual included weighing ourselves on a regular basis, talking about how to lose weight in my case, and learning how to eat better even though money was tight at home. During my three-year stint with Bill I lost forty-five pounds! I still remember him saying to me, "Bill, you could be a good basketball player, but we need to work on slimming you down so you can move faster." It wasn't *me* doing it on my own; it was *us* working on my weight loss and diet together. Bill also wanted to know all about our family lives, the good and the bad, our schooling, and what mischief we were creating for ourselves. We trusted him and could talk about personal things we usually kept to ourselves.

Bill also let us know about himself. He talked about his own late start going to college after his armed service stint, marrying early, and having three kids at home and his day job with kids with disabilities. He invited us to his home for special occasions, and we saw firsthand what life was like in a home where people were not living paycheck to paycheck. Many of us gym rats, as we were called, found in Bill an adult mentor whom we wanted to be like. It was no surprise that many of us found our way into teaching and coaching because of his quiet and steady influence. I learned the important lesson that one skilled adult can indeed intervene to help many teens by being present in their lives and teaching them that a healthier and more successful lifestyle is possible, within their reach. Bill was a gift for me and my peers at a time in our lives when we needed a positive role model who stressed that we had worth and value and that we could contribute to the world in our own unique way. We had something to offer others. Bill, in a real sense, helped raise me and taught me about the adult world along with my mother and father, who welcomed Bill's presence in my life. They saw the difference he made in me, a difference they alone could not make. We were all in it together.

Ervin Fieger entered my life in grade ten. Fieger was the boys' physical education teacher and basketball coach. He, like Bill, was a veteran and had entered the teaching profession in his early thirties. He was the model of a fit, health, energetic physical education teacher and coach. He was always on time, prepared, and expecting students to be involved. I never saw him "just throw out the ball" and sit on the sidelines until the period ended. He was also a caring and temperate educator who was interested in having his students enjoy the gym and the activities it offered. Coach Fieger was the same way coaching basketball. He was interested in developing winning teams, which he did, but he also wanted his players to learn about teamwork and sharing the ball with others, to be patient and accepting when games went badly, and to show respect for the other team. He was into personal and health development for his players, stressing the need to be on time, rested, eating a healthy diet (which he described for us), and allowing no put-downs of players on our team or the opposing team. He said, "Avoid reading your press clippings. Things can change quickly for would-be stars." He also had a calming "I know we can succeed here" approach in close contests; he wasn't a yeller, a screamer, or the type to respond with anger when the referees seemed to make bad calls.

In the fall of tenth grade Bill Carmichael urged me to go out for the junior varsity basketball team. He felt that I was ready to earn a spot. In fact, Fieger approached me in the fall and asked me to try out. He too suggested I try to lose some weight as it might help me earn a spot on the team. I did make the team but at first felt overwhelmed by the other players, all of whom came from Hingham and had played together through the early grades and junior high. Fieger seemed to understand my feeling out of the loop and constantly tried to work me into the team, stressing that my height could help the team's defense and offensive rebounding.

With Fieger's intervention, along with Bill Carmichael's ongoing guidance, I continued to lose weight and made the starting five in my junior and senior years. I was not a star player. I had no future as a college player. But I had found another home and mentor/parent figure in Ervin Fieger and the basketball team. That home helped me establish strong personal ties with Hingham kids, and I became more involved in school social activities and became a much-improved academic student after failing most of my classes in ninth grade.

Finding a home in school and an adult mentor who can play some of the roles missing in one's home life can serve to promote pride in oneself, lead to improvement in health and academics, and assist in the search for a healthy and rewarding lifestyle and one's place in the world.

Coach Ward Donner also was a big influence in my continued weight loss and my path to becoming fit. Donner was the head coach of football, basketball, and baseball at Thayer Academy in Braintree, Massachusetts. While most of my Hull peers joined the Army, Air Force, or Marines after graduation, I decided to continue my studies at Thayer, a nearby day college preparatory school. This was my next step in discovering I could fit in with achieving students from so-called good families who lived in the wealthy suburbs of Boston. At Thayer I found other athletes from poor areas who were post-grad students trying to use athletics as a stepping-stone to college scholarships. But more importantly I found in Ward Donner a real teacher.

Donner was the school's head administrator and disciplinarian as well as coach. He had attended an Ivy League college, where he excelled in sports and academics. He had come to Thayer as a young teacher and coach and stayed on to establish himself as a beloved educator, mentor, and coach for the many Thayer grads who moved on to college and professional successes. He was also a gentleman's gentleman, dressed in Brooks Brothers shirts, jacket, pants, socks, and shoes, with a different striped tie each day. He was Mr. Ivy League. He had a quiet but caring demeanor, never saying too much while coaching and disciplining students but always a good listener, available and willing to offer both praise and tempered criticism in sports and academics and expecting the best from his students and players.

Ward Donner, like Bill Carmichael and Ervin Fieger, helped me to fit in. I played basketball and baseball for him. He stressed physical and mental preparation, urging a daily running and workout regimen. Donner's teams played in a college-prep league that took us to private day and boarding schools all over New England. It was a real eye-opener for a once-overweight teen from Hull who had been on the road to perhaps dropping out of high school and at risk for a shortened lifespan like the men in his neighborhood. Now I was on the road to visiting and competing against, as Donner said, the best-prepared and brightest students in the world. I was fit, "in the club," as the saying goes, and a contender. It is no wonder that I decided during my Thayer experience that I wanted a career as an educator, to be like Carmichael, Fieger, and Donner. I wanted to do for others what they had done for me. I had found my niche. So I know something about the need for physical education teachers and coaches to intervene with overweight and obese students because I am a successful case study and disciple of what intervention can bring.

Not every teen is as fortunate as I was, to have skilled educators such as Carmichael, Fieger, and Donner in their corner, educators who saw it as part of their job to address the health and well-being of students like Bill Fibkins. Clearly the effort to address teen obesity will require training and empowering many more such educators. As a nation we can no longer afford to support physical education teachers and programs that have a practice of focusing all their efforts on athletic teams that involve only a small percentage of students and ignore the great potential that school gym classes have to improve the fitness of all students. Using gym classes to simply "throw out the ball and let the kids play" doesn't cut it in a society where kids are unfit. We need to elevate the role of physical activity in physical education programs.

Medical writer Lindsey Tanner spells out the critical need for schools to provide increased opportunities for teens to engage in rigorous physical activity. She cites research indicating that a third of U.S. teens would flunk a treadmill fitness test, meaning that more than 7 million youngsters could face higher risks of heart disease later in life. Dr. David Ludwig, director of the obesity program at Children's Hospital in Boston, says the research, while surprising given previous research findings that about 16% of U.S. schoolchildren are seriously overweight, is still "very concerning and shows that at a time in life when adolescents and young adults should be at peak levels of fitness, there's in fact a very high prevalence of low fitness."[3] The research, an analysis of nationally representative data from government health surveys by Northwestern University researchers, found that 24% of girls and boys ages twelve to nineteen showed a poor level of cardiovascular fitness on an eight-minute treadmill test. Teens and adults with poor fitness were two to four times more likely to be overweight and obese than those considered moderately or highly fit, the study found. Waist size, cholesterol levels, and blood pressure were also higher in those in the low fitness category. Mercedes Carnethon, the lead author of the research, said, "While adolescents aren't at risk for heart diseases in the short term, this research data has important implications for the long-term health of youth in the United States."[4]

According to medical writer Paul Simao, these unhealthy fitness patterns follow many teens into adult life. Most U.S. adults failed to exercise at the minimum recommended level in 2003, according to a federal government study released on December 1, 2005. Only 45.9% of those ages eighteen and over met the U.S. government's recommendation of at least thirty minutes of brisk walking or other moderate exercise five days a week or at least twenty minutes of vigorous exercise three days a week.[5]

Dr. David Satcher, former surgeon general of the United States, suggests that the healthy eating and physical activity experience of children and teens in our schools plays a critical role in improving their health. Satcher says, "We must prime our children academically, but academic success will be moot if a student does not realize her or his potential because of poor health and/or an abbreviated life." Satcher argues that providing more time for increased physical activity leads to increased academic test scores. He advises, "We can no longer afford to cut physical education and good nutrition in our schools; doing so may be penny-wise, but it is literally pound foolish. I look to the schools as a powerful force for change."[6] There can be no disagreement that what students experience each day in their schools does play an important role in shaping their long-term health, for good or for bad. As Satcher says, the money schools invest in nutrition and physical educations programs will be a "down payment" that ultimately saves lives, a down payment that does not have to be just monetary. It can be in the form of awareness in turning around the lives of overweight and obese teens.

Clearly, as John P. Allegrante, president of the National Center for Health Education, observes, physical activity in the school can boost self-discipline, reduce stress, strengthen peer relationships, enhance self-confidence and self-esteem, and improve mental alertness. Students with health problems are not as ready or able to learn. Allegrante cites a study of hundreds of thousands of fifth, seventh, and ninth graders conducted in 2002 by the California Department of Education that offers the most convincing anecdotal support for this idea. Physically fit youngsters in the study posted significantly higher scores on math and reading tests. Allegrante suggests that American schools should be doing much more to engage students in vigorous physical activity than they do now. He says that more than a third of young people in grades nine through twelve do not regularly engage in vigorous physical activity and more than 10% get no physical activity at all. Allegrante offers his analysis, saying, "As long as schools are tightening their belts instead of their students' waistlines, I'm afraid every child will be left behind."[7]

Allegrante's observations are supported by researchers at the University of North Carolina at Chapel Hill, who say they have found concrete evidence to back up what child-health experts have known intuitively for years: students who do not participate in regular physical education or community recreation programs are far more likely to become couch potatoes.[8] According to writer Kathleen Kennedy Manzo, while the North Carolina data support a critical role for physical education in school, the researchers found that the overwhelming majority of middle and high school students are not enrolled in PE courses. As Manzo points out, this kind of inactivity has been found to put children and adults at greater risk of obesity and serious health problems.[9] The research data point out that despite the marked and significant impact of participation in school PE programs on physical activity patterns of U.S. adolescents, few adolescents participated in such programs.[10]

The report called for national-level strategies that include attention to school PE and community recreation programs, particularly for those segments of the U.S. population without access to resources and opportunities that allow participation in physical activity. The researchers studied data on nearly 18,000 middle and high school students. Among the nationally represented sample, eight in ten students reported that they were not enrolled in PE courses. One of the authors of the report, Penny Gordon-Larson, a postdoctoral fellow in multidisciplinary nutrition studies at the University of North Carolina, says, "PE really fills an important role in increasing activity among American kids. For a lot of low income families who don't have resources in their neighborhoods, the school is available to all kids, and physical education can equalize access so that all kids have resources to be active."[11]

While the University of North Carolina report suggests there is much work to be done to bring about quality physical education for every student, I believe the epidemic of teen obesity is serving to bring about national-level strategies that include attention to improving school physical education programs. The debate over how best to address teen obesity has served to create an increased awareness among educators, parents, and community leaders that the schools are ideally suited to offer many existing and potential opportunities to engage students in healthy eating and physical activity. As David Satcher suggests, "We must prime our children academically, but academic success will be moot if a student does not realize her or his potential because of poor health and/or an abbreviated life."

Backed by a national movement, physical education programs are increasingly being seen as vital components in reducing teen obesity and related health problems, increasing teens' academic success, and providing them with healthy lifestyle skills that can lead to a successful and healthy life, a life in which they can play an active role, contribute, and be a contender like the young Bill Fibkins. Physical education teachers are increasingly being seen as skilled professionals who play an important role in intervening to help unhealthy teens. With the emergence of the obesity epidemic, they are no longer relegated to a role in the school hierarchy where they historically have been looked down upon by many academic teachers, students, and community members—unless they have a winning sports team.

It's no wonder that they have gravitated toward coaching and the esteem that comes their way with a winning season. For many physical education teachers, coaching, with all its extra time, stress, and conflicts, has been the only way to achieve professional parity and be valued by academic subject teachers. Often they were hired as coaches to fill a need or vacancy. Teaching physical education was a secondary role. This was particularly true when the Title IX law came into being in the early 1970s, a law that required the speedy hiring of many coaches to lead the young women's athletic teams. The obesity epidemic has provided a way they can now be valued for their teaching skills as well as their coaching skills.

The teaching role for physical educators is also beginning to gather support from parents in addition to leading health officials such as David Satcher. A National Association for Sports and Physical Education (NASPE) press release states that parents' overwhelming support for not wanting to reduce their children's physical education time allotment to provide more academic classes is one more testament to the role of physical education classes in helping children become healthy, physically active adults.[12] The press release was in response to the results of a survey released by the American Obesity Association in September 2000, which strongly opposed cutting back on physical education classes. In the spring of 2000 NASPE released its own parent survey that complements the one conducted by the American Obesity Association. Among parents with children in elementary, middle, and high school, 81% want their kids to receive daily physical education classes, but only 44% percent report that the children are receiving them.[13]

Dr. Marybell Avery, NASPE president and curriculum specialist for health and physical education in the Lincoln, Nebraska, public schools, said in the press release,

Evidence mounts daily for the importance of quality physical education programs from the US Surgeon General and other medical and health experts. Unfortunately many school districts are not providing these opportunities. According to NASPE's Shape of the Nation survey, in thirty-seven states the majority of physical education classes are taught by classroom teachers and the majority of high school students take physical education for only one year between ninth and twelfth grades. NASPE recommends 150 minutes a week for elementary and 225 minutes per week for secondary students. In addition, physical education classes need to have adequate equipment and facilities so that every child can participate.[14]

I believe the current national debate about teen obesity and the awareness that health and fitness do influence learning will spur parents, educators, and community members into action, as was the case in changing the school lunch program at East Hampton Middle School. Many parents are educating themselves about the importance of physical activity for their children and reading information such as the United States Department of Human Services report "Physical Activity Fundamental to Preventing Diseases," which was issued in June 2002. The report advocates regular physical activity for students and suggests that such activity plays an important role in students' staying in school and having good conduct and high academic achievement, as well as developing skills such as teamwork, self-discipline, sportsmanship, leadership, and socialization. Moreover, the report suggests that physical activity reduces morbidity and mortality from health and mental health disorders.[15] As noted above, 81% of parents in the NASPE study want daily physical education classes. Many of these parents are showing up at school board meetings and demanding change.

As seen in East Hampton, grassroots political action by students and parents supported by risk-taking teachers and administrators can hasten the shift to a new model of health and physical education. This is represented by educators such as Ginny Reale, an educator whose primary responsibility is being a health and physical education teacher, who promote and implement a wellness philosophy among students, staff, and parents. This intervention process can increase awareness among students and parents and can lead to political advocacy that can be translated into critical votes for or against local school budgets and bring about changes in school lunch programs that can benefit the health and well-being of students.

Parent awareness and advocacy can also challenge education leaders such as John R. Woolums, director of governmental relations for the Maryland Association of Boards of Education. According to writer Christian Davenport, Woolums said, "Students already have many demands on their time and forcing them to exercise would only cut away from academics. We really barely have time for English, language arts, math and the core components." Woolums was responding to a bill that would make it mandatory for all Maryland school children to get five hours of exercise a week because Maryland health officials are increasingly concerned about overweight children and the illnesses that obesity can lead to. Woolums was urging a Maryland House of Delegates committee not to pass the measure. The sponsor of the measure, state delegate Joan F. Stern, said, "We're at a point with obesity where we were with tobacco twenty years ago, when we didn't understand the extent of the problem."[16]

As I document in this book, we are gradually beginning to understand the problem of teens being overweight or obese and the associated health risks of developing long-term illnesses such as diabetes, heart disease, and so forth. We do know that there are new physical education intervention models that are successful in helping teens become fit and healthy. Data about these models need to be widely shared among national, state, and local groups of educators, parents, students, and community members so they will be well informed and aware of what can work to reduce teen overweight and obesity in our schools.

The National Alliance for Nutrition and Activity (NANA) "Model Local School Wellness Policies on Physical Activity and Nutrition" report offers a comprehensive model for the new physical education program that needs to be developed in the schools. The report recommends that all students in grades K–12, including students with disabilities or special health-care needs and those in alternative settings, receive daily physical education (or its equivalent of 150 minutes per week for elementary students and 225 minutes per week for middle and high school students) for the entire school year. All physical education classes will be taught by a certified physical education teacher. Students' involvement in other physical activities (i.e., interscholastic or intramural sports) may not be substituted for meeting the physical education requirement. Students must spend at least 50% of physical education class time in moderate to vigorous physical activity. Schools should discourage extended periods of inactivity, such as are required for mandatory testing, by offering periodic breaks. Schools should also offer physical activity opportunities before and after school, such as physical activity clubs and intramural programs as well as interscholastic sports programs.[17]

What is needed now are concrete examples of how individual schools, such as Moorhead High, have succeeded in implementing some of the components of the new physical education models advocated for in local wellness policies. I believe the physical education program at Madison Junior High in Naperville, Illinois, offers such an example and offers important lessons on how education leaders can make the visions of increased physical activity for students that are recommended in local wellness policies a reality. Here is the Madison Junior High story.

The new PE curriculum is beginning to take hold in many schools thanks to the leadership of forward-thinking educators such as Phil Lawler, physical education coordinator at Madison Junior High in Naperville, Illinois. Reporter Roberta Furger describes how Lawler has used high-tech tools to help bring a healthier, more balanced approach to physical education. Furger observes that from the heart-rate monitors that students wear during their weekly twelve-minute run/walk to a comprehensive computer-based fitness station where students measure everything from strength and flexibility to cholesterol levels, Madison Junior High has embraced the use of state-of-the-art tools to support the physical health and education of adolescent students. Included among Madison's unique PE facility are a complete fitness center, a rock-climbing wall, and a series of computer-enabled fitness test stations where students create a total health portfolio that will eventually follow them from sixth grade through high school graduation.[18]

Furger's observations are also supported in more detail by WTTW-Chicago reporter Elizabeth Brackett, who states that 30% of the schools in Illinois have new physical education programs, many of which look like local health clubs. Brackett suggests that physical education is more than volleyball and competitive sports, as in the past. Brackett also points out the value of the "new PE" pioneered at schools such as Madison Junior High. For example, physical education students at the school spend their forty-minute gym period scaling down walls, running on treadmills, and using weight machines.[19] But innovative "new PE" and health programs do not happen without leadership. As in East Hampton, where wellness changes were led by teacher Ginny Reale, the new physical education model that emerged in Naperville was led by Phil Lawler, a forward-thinking and acting educator.

Change does require a vision, risk taking, and sales promotion skills by educators like Reale and Lawler to get administrators, staff, students, parents, and community members on board. Data are needed to convince various constituencies that change is necessary. For example, when Lawler first began to share his vision to make a major shift in the school's physical education philosophy, he used data from research by cardiologist Vincent Bufalino to support the change. Bufalino had measured the cholesterol levels of 5,000 children ages five to seventeen in Du Page County and found that an astonishing 35–40% had high cholesterol. Lawler used the data as a major argument for change in the physical education program at Madison Junior High and other district and area schools. He formed a partnership with Bufalino, who reviewed the data and found that it was not so much genetic but that fast-food restaurant use and lack of exercise were the two biggest predictors of whether kids had high cholesterol or not.[20]

Clearly Lawler's partnership with Bufalino was an excellent leadership strategy, a strategy that provided him with creditable data that he could bring to school, parent, and community leaders and also gave him a platform for change. Bufalino became a big booster of Lawler's program. And it appears that Lawler understood that he had to sell his vision to business, parent, and community leaders who would be in a position to offer additional resources.

Brackett reports that Lawler found support for the new physical education movement from Chicago-based Wilson Sporting Goods

Company, whose president Jim Baugh says, "You have to condition people. Just like you're teaching kids how to read and write or arithmetic, you have to teach them how to develop an active lifestyle."[21] Baugh founded PE for Life, a national advocacy group to promote funding for daily physical education programs across the country. Efforts by PE for Life and other lobbying groups have resulted in $50 million in grants to upgrade physical education programs in a recently passed education appropriations bill.[22]

However, while Lawler had the support of business leaders like Jim Baugh, he also had to beat a steady path to parents and community members in order to sell his vision, break down resistance, elicit financial and political support, and solicit donations such as equipment. Leaders with vision need to attend many coffee klatches, PTA and community meetings, and dinners at organizations such as the Lions Club. Selling one's vision is very much like running for political office—lots of chicken dinners, cold coffee, and late-night and early-morning meetings.

Reporter Kevin V. Johnson says that Phil Lawler wheels and deals to get the equipment his students need. When PE money dried up, he argued that money for more heart monitors should come from the technology budget. Regular coffee klatches with parents helped lay the groundwork for donations when he needed $14,000 to build a rock-climbing wall. He scoured classified ads for used weight machines. A local rehab and sports performance clinic loaned its personnel to operate muscle and stress-testing machines so Lawler could create an annually updated fitness record for each student, showing muscle strength, cardiovascular condition, and cholesterol levels. Lawler is now looking for a corporation to finance a ten-to-twenty-year tracking study that will chart the long-term value of the "New PE" Program.[23] And Lawler has the energy to carry out his vision. As the reader knows, there are many good ideas for education reform. However, making these good ideas into reality not only takes vision but also takes the ability to work hard and have a high level of energy that can sustain the Lawlers of the world when push comes to shove in change efforts.

Jerry Virgo, former principal of Madison Junior High, says, "Lawler is a very energetic person. He's sold on PE and has endless enthusiasm for what he is doing."[24] And as Johnson reports, "Lawler practices what he preaches, spending thirty minutes in the zone on his treadmill each morning."[25] He is fit for the task.

Roberta Furger reports that Lawler's efforts have earned him a national reputation,[26] and he uses his platform to remind educators,

> New PE programs must show measurable results just as academic programs are measured by test score results. At Madison, a fitness profile is developed for each student that includes the wearing of heart-rate monitors so teachers and students can measure their effort level. The results are downloaded after class and become a part of the student's fitness profile. Lawler says "the monitors taught me that even slow-moving students may be exercising at their maximum level of effort. In the old days everything was, let's run a mile and if you can't run a mile in under eight minutes, you're a failure. Well, how many people in this country were turned off to exercise by those standards? Well, technology proved that our judgment was wrong. We have learned to personalize it and give kids credit for what they do."[27]

Lawler is also able to make the important connection between the value of the daily delivery of physical education and increased academic performance. He reports that the school finished number one in the world in science and sixth in math on the Tims test. Lawler states, "We truly feel we were a contributing factor to these test scores with the brain research that says physical activity affects the brain."[28]

As the "Physical Activity Fundamental to Preventing Disease" research cited above suggests, physical activity may stimulate new brain cells that enhance memory and learning. Lawler is not hesitant to challenge the old physical education model that focused mainly on coaching interscholastic sports and viewed teaching gym class as a necessary evil that offered only the benefit of scouting future varsity athletes. As Furger says of the old physical education model, many teens who participated in gym were left with a lifetime of bad memories like being picked last for basketball scrimmage or being ridiculed by teachers and fellow students for being too weak or slow.[29] And, I would add, too fat.

In his interview with Brackett, Lawler says,

It used to be that we were meeting the needs of about thirty or forty percent of our population. Those were the athletes. And the others were brought along. They were forced to take what we were offering, but really saw no value in it, really didn't enjoy it. They dreaded gym class with its focus on team sports. The "old PE" model attended to skills many kids won't be using as adults and has left many of them on the sideline.[30]

A letter from a parent, Mike Reynolds, to Lawler vividly demonstrates the negative impact of the "old PE" on him:

Kudos to your PE program. In junior high and high school I was one of the slow kids. I was not obese, just plain slow. I remember my PE teacher shouting when it was my turn to run the 100-yard dash, "Oh, Reynolds is up, someone get me a calendar to time him!" I learned to hate PE through high school and college. I "let myself go" physically, hating to participate in sports, and that turned into hatred for exercise. When I was 28, and saw what I had become, and I saw another out-of-shape friend suffer a heart attack at 32, I was motivated to exercise, bring my blood pressure to normal, lose 70 pounds back to my normal weight, and have learned to enjoy exercise. I am 31 now, doing well, and in the best shape of my life. I wish I was this way all my life. I believe if I, and others like me, participated in a program such as the one at Madison, we would not have had to suffer the ridicule in school, and most importantly having to suffer life in an out-of-shape body, wondering if your heart can make it to 40. I hope my children will have the privilege of participating in a Physical Education program similar to the one at Madison.[31]

Mike Reynolds's story of ridicule, hatred of physical education and sports, and visions of a heart attack by age forty and a shortened lifespan all began in a gym class supposedly offered to improve health and well-being. It clearly points out the experience of many slow, overweight, obese, and poorly coordinated teens in the "old PE" gym classes. The experience clearly had the opposite effect from "improving health and well-being" for Reynolds.

Reynolds shouldn't have had to wait until he reached the age of twenty-eight to become healthier. As Dr. Bufalino told Elizabeth Brackett, "If we don't teach kids to exercise early, we're not going to get them to do it when they're 40 or 50, when I see them and they're ready for their bypass surgery. And we have to put a scar on their chest to convince them they should start exercising. Something is wrong with that."[32] It's hard-hitting advice. As a teenager Mike Reynolds clearly could have benefited from involvement with physical education teachers such as Moorhead High's Tony Jankowski and Marge Edgar, Ginny Reale, Bill Carmichael, Ervin Fieger, Ward Donner, and Phil Lawler.

As ABC reporter Linda Yu points out, Naperville Central High School students Jennifer Mayor and Jessica Wolfrum are fortunate teens who have benefited from Lawler's "new PE" in Naperville. Mayor says that as a freshman she was afraid of gym class and nonathletic. "Being heavy was really hard. I was lazy, sick as a kid, taking prednisone. No self-esteem. No confidence." Jennifer learned to set goals for herself daily in gym class, and as she lost forty pounds, she found confidence that she could achieve these goals. She is now in college. "Once you see that you can take something and change it. I'm in school now, studying business. I don't just want to be a manager. I want to be a CEO." Jessica Wolfrum told Linda Yu that the "new PE" has increased her self-confidence. She was a shy, quiet freshman. Achieving physical milestones makes her a leader. "You surprise yourself. You don't expect something of yourself and then you do it and then you ask, 'What else can I do?' You unleash something inside you. You didn't know you were so strong."[33]

Reporter Kevin V. Johnson also describes an example of Lawler's positive impact on students. As a Northwestern University freshman in 2003, former student Nadine Youssef credited Lawler and the "new PE" with changing her attitude toward exercise. She says,

I was never really in sports, or dedicated to athletics. But with the heart monitor I knew I was working just as hard as the kids in track and gym who were running six-minute miles, even if they lapped me. I didn't dread going to gym because I knew I wouldn't be embarrassed.

And you always enjoy the things you succeed at. The program definitely made me aware of the importance of being healthy and able to
go the distance.[34]

As Lawler told reporter Roberta Furger, "What it all boils down to
is information. We want to provide students with the tools and the
information they need to live healthy, active lives."[35] And, I would
add, we need to provide the same tools for school staff and parents.
Clearly former Naperville students Jennifer Mayor, Jessica Wolfrum,
and Nadine Youssef received the tools and information they needed
to live healthy, active lives. Lawler provides an excellent model on
how educators can put "physical" back into physical education and
teach students like Mike Reynolds how to lead healthy, active lives,
not be ridiculed and threatened by educators and programs that are
supposed to help them.

Lawler's groundbreaking work is critically important as it offers a
model other school wellness teams can replicate or adopt components from that fit their budget and needs. Susan Okie, MD, puts the
importance of Lawler's work in its proper context when she reports
that kids get between 20% and 40% of their total physical activity at
school.[36] School gym classes and recess provide the only strenuous
exercise many U.S. children get during the week. Yet studies suggest
that at most schools the minutes children actually spend in vigorous
activity are few indeed. Trained observers watching physical education classes found that students engaged in only about three minutes of moderate to vigorous exercise per class.[37]

Lawler's work also points out the importance of physical education
for secondary school students. Okie says that as children move from
childhood into adolescence, starting at about age ten, physical activity levels for both sexes, especially for girls, begin to decline. Decreased emphasis on PE classes after elementary school probably
contributes to part of the reduction. About half of U.S. schools require physical education for students in grades one through five, but
this percentage drops off steeply in the higher grades. Fewer than
10% of high schools require physical education for students in grades

ten through twelve, even though PE programs have been shown to have a strong impact on activity levels in this age group.[38]

Okie also suggests that along with declining overall activity levels, adolescents of both sexes participate in fewer physically active leisure-time activities such as basketball, bicycling, softball, running, and aerobics as they get older. She says this decline in leisure activity could be related to academic pressure, exclusion from competitive sports programs, lack of parental support, or the lure of sedentary forms of entertainment such as television and computer games.[39]

Addressing the negative aspects of competitive sports programs, Okie cites research by James F. Sallis, a professor of psychology at San Diego State University, that suggests that high school sports programs, with their emphasis on competitiveness and athletic prowess, take money away from physical education programs and paradoxically discourage many teenagers from remaining active. Sallis says, "There's this pyramid, especially as kids get older. If they're not the athletic elite, they are invited out of the athletic program and excluded. We think that this policy to pursue competition and winning, instead of promoting health in these kids, is actually contributing to the decline in activity with age. The opportunities that are available to kids as they get older are diminished by design."[40]

As medical writer Lindsey Tanner reports, participating in competitive athletics can provide its own health risks for teenagers, including injuries that can have long-term medical implications and in some cases are life-threatening. In addition to injuries such as concussions and broken bones, there are also health risks that occur in training practice in some sports. Tanner cites a policy statement from the American Academy of Pediatrics that warned, "Weight loss accompanied by over-exercising, excessive dieting, using rubber suits, steam baths or saunas should be prohibited for all young athletes. So should diet pills, nutritional supplements and diuretics and no weight loss plan for athletic purposes should be used before ninth grade." The policy statement applies to youngsters in sports where leanness or strength is emphasized, including wrestling, body-building, gymnastics, football, figure skating, and cheerleading. As the policy states, these are sports in which coaches may encourage unhealthy weight management practices that can lead to problems, including eating disorders, dehydration, heat stress, and gaining too much fat instead of muscle, which can lead to cardiovascular problems. Wrestlers are especially prone to trying dangerous weight-loss methods as they are often encouraged to compete in the lowest possible weight class.[41]

Lawler's efforts appear to be aimed at demonstrating that the "new PE" offers the opportunity for schools to improve the health of students. While he doesn't come out with strong attacks on the "old PE" model with its emphasis on winning athletic teams, his efforts are clearly causing administrators, physical education teachers, and parents to rethink what constitutes "physical activity" in the schools and ask the question, "Are the students receiving their share?" The "old PE" bastions may not be crumbling, but the winning-games philosophy that supports the "old PE" is being challenged.

Lawler's efforts to promote the "new PE" are succeeding. He is demonstrating that physical education is needed by students at the secondary level, that students other than, as Sallis says, the "athletic elite" need opportunities for vigorous exercise without the health risks involved in competitive athletics, that the vital health indicators of students, such as cholesterol and blood pressure levels, should be monitored, that the schools should tap into health and medical resources such as Dr. Bufalino, and that each student should have a fitness profile and fitness report. Lawler has a new vision, and it appears that he is delivering in spades.

There are many lessons that school leaders and wellness team members can learn from the Naperville experiment as they try to implement local policies to improve nutrition and physical activity for students. As a student of education-reform efforts, I see one lesson that stands out for me and that I believe will require early attention. That lesson is that while schools can embrace the written recommendations of such policies, the implementation stage that soon follows will require the leadership of savvy and committed educators like Phil Lawler and Ginny Reale, educators who have a vision, are able to articulate that vision and share it with a variety of constituencies, are able to enlist the support of these constituencies and get them on board the change effort, can share the successes of the change effort so that many individuals and groups are affirmed for their participation, are able to weather setbacks and failures that are inevitable and manage to change course, are physically and emotionally prepared to lead the change process, and are willing to remain in a leadership role and not move on until the project has support and becomes a recognized part of the school district's curriculum.

Too often leaders become national and state "stars" and become overly involved in self-promotion at conferences and/or spend too much time assisting and consulting with other districts with the result being that the program they developed loses its momentum as the leader with vision moves on and leaves the program to drift, abandoned because of the lure of professional success elsewhere.

NOTES

1. Peter C. Beller, "Boycott or No, Students Get Results," *New York Times*, 10 Apr. 2005, http://query.nytimes.com/gst/fullpage.html?res=9C01E2DC1 63EF933A25757C0A9639C8 (accessed 5 May 2005).

2. Kim Severson, "Eating, Writing and 'Rithmetic: Harlem Pupils Meet Swiss Chard," *New York Times*, 9 Sept. 2005, B5.

3. Lindsey Tanner, "Many Teens Would Flunk Treadmill Test," Associated Press, 20 Dec. 2005, http://www.yahoo.com/s/ap/20051220/ ap_on_he_me/fit_unfit_kids (accessed 21 Dec. 2005).

4. Tanner, "Many Teens."

5. Paul Simao, "Many Americans Choose Couch Over Treadmill," Reuters, 1 Dec. 2005, http://www.yahoo.com/s/nm/20051201/us_nm/ exercise_dc (accessed 21 Dec. 2005).

6. David Satcher, "Pound-Foolish," *Education Week*, 16 Oct. 2002, http://www.edweek.org/ew/articles/2002/10/16/07satcher.h22.html (accessed 25 May 2005).

7. John P. Allegrante, "Unfit to Learn," *Education Week*, 1 Dec. 2004, http://www.edweek.org/ew/articles/2004/12/01/14allegrante.h24.html (accessed 25 May 2005).

8. Kathleen Kennedy Manzo, "PE Promotes Active Lifestyle Among Adolescents, Study Finds," *Education Week*, 14 June 2000, http://www.edweek.org/ew/articles/2000/06/14/40obese.h19? (accessed 25 May 2005).

9. Kennedy Manzo, "PE Promotes Active Lifestyle."

10. Kennedy Manzo, "PE Promotes Active Lifestyle."

11. Kennedy Manzo, "PE Promotes Active Lifestyle."

12. National Association for Sports and Physical Education (NASPE), "Physical Educators Buoyant Over Parents Support in American Obesity Association Survey," NASPE press release, 13 Dec. 2000.

13. NASPE, "Physical Educators Buoyant."

14. NASPE, "Physical Educators Buoyant."

15. United States Department of Health and Human Services, "Physical Activity Fundamental to Preventing Diseases," 20 June 2002, http://aspe.hhs.gov/health/reports/physicalactivity/index.shtml (accessed 22 June 2005).

16. Christine Davenport, "Student Obesity Targeted," *Washington Post*, 11 Feb. 2004, http://www.washingtonpost.com/ac2/wp-dyn/A30235-2004 Feb10? (accessed 3 Nov. 2004).

17. National Alliance for Nutrition and Activity (NANA), "Model Local School Wellness Policies on Physical Activity and Nutrition," Center for Science in the Public Interest, Mar. 2005, http://www.schoolwellnesspolicies.org (accessed 2 June 2005), 1–26.

18. Roberta Furger, "The New P.E. Curriculum," edutopia, 1 Aug. 2001, http://www.edutopia.org/php/article.php?id=Art_838 (accessed 27 June 2005).

19. Elizabeth Brackett, "Fit for Life," Online NewsHour, 22 Mar. 2002, http://www.pbs.org/newshour/bbeducation/jan-june02/pe_3-22.html (accessed 27 June 2005).

20. Brackett, "Fit for Life."

21. Brackett, "Fit for Life."

22. Brackett, "Fit for Life."

23. Kevin V. Johnson, "New P.E. Teacher Takes Students to the Max: Every Activity Stresses Cardiovascular Fitness," *USA Today*, 13 Jan. 2003, http://www.usatoday.com/usatonline/200030113/4773184s.htm (accessed 27 June 2005).

24. Johnson, "New P.E. Teacher."

25. Johnson, "New P.E. Teacher."

26. Furger, "The New P.E. Curriculum."

27. Brackett, "Fit for Life."

28. Brackett, "Fit for Life."

29. Furger, "The New P.E. Curriculum."

30. Brackett, "Fit for Life."

31. Madison Junior High School, "PE Forum: Advocacy," letter to staff and parents from administrator Steve Jeffries, 1 June 2001, http://www.ncusd203.org/madisonnewpe-letters.html (accessed 3 June 2005).

32. Brackett, "Fit for Life."

33. Linda Yu, "Learner for Life: 'New PE,'" ABC.com, 3 Dec. 2003, http://abclocal.go.com/wls/news/specialsegments_Nov02/020903_ss_Learner.html (accessed 27 June 2005).

34. Johnson, "New P.E. Teacher."

35. Furger, "The New P.E. Curriculum."

36. Susan Okie, *Fed Up! Winning the War Against Childhood Obesity* (Washington, DC: Joseph Henry Press, 2005), 122.

37. Okie, *Fed Up!* 122.

38. Okie, *Fed Up!* 123.

39. Okie, *Fed Up!* 123–24.

40. Okie, *Fed Up!* 124–25.

41. Lindsey Tanner, "Young Athletes at Risk Over Weight-Control," Associated Press, 12 Dec. 2005, http://news.yahoo.com/s/ap/20051205/ap_on_he_me/fit_child_athletes_weight (accessed 5 Dec. 2005).

6

UTILIZING THE CIRCLE OF WELLNESS TO IMPROVE NUTRITION AND PHYSICAL ACTIVITY FOR STUDENTS

I believe the data and case studies identified in this book offer evidence that school wellness teams need a multicomponent model that includes ten strategies necessary to implement a successful local wellness policy to improve student nutrition and activity and address health issues such as overweight and obesity. I call this model the Circle of Wellness model. While this model includes three major approaches recommended by researchers such as Susan Okie, activists, and parents trying to combat the obesity epidemic through schools, it also offers new approaches based on my own experience in the schools. The three major approaches advocated by Okie and others are as follows:

1. Improve and expand physical education programs or find additional ways of incorporating physical education into the school day.
2. Stop schools from selling foods and beverages high in calories and low in nutrients and try to ensure that all meals, snacks, and drinks available in the school are healthy.
3. Get schools to adopt curricula that teach the importance of good diet and daily physical activity, curricula that also motivate students to try out and adopt new health habits.[1]

My Circle of Wellness model also includes important components such as school wellness team leadership; involvement of parents and community health, mental health, and recreation organizations as partners; wellness programs for staff that are similar to the services offered to students; and increased use of technology to monitor important health indicators for students and staff, with the same monitoring opportunities available for parents after school hours. Here are the necessary components in the Circle of Wellness model:

1. Wellness team efforts need leaders such as Al Morris, Ginny Reale, and Phil Lawler who have a vision for change and can rally the many constituencies in the school and community. The efforts of these leaders represent what is possible utilizing new approaches to nutrition and the "new PE" to improve physical activity. Wellness teams need enthusiastic leaders who are doers, can deliver programs, and have the will to win the battle for improved health for our children. They need educators who will stay the course and continue to beat the drum for the wellness program and develop new strategies and programs as new needs arise. Successful wellness programs, like other examples of education reform success stories, don't stay the same over time. They require constant shoring up and changes of course to remain current. Otherwise, as I have observed many times, successful programs slowly lose their value and political clout. Susan Okie addresses the personnel and resources needed in a successful education project by saying, "Leadership, a sense of purpose, clear educational principles, passionate and energetic teachers, adequate space and resources, involvement by parents and by the local community, the same qualities a school needs to effectively teach reading and math, are what it needs to teach children how to be healthy."[2]

2. The wellness team efforts need to be viewed as honest and genuine, not as a public relations blitz that glosses over inadequacies in wellness programs. Simply put, educators can't sim-

ply talk about the need for improved nutrition and physical activity and then fail to deliver on what was promised. A sense of hypocrisy will develop if wellness teams promote the value of vigorous physical activity but PE teachers fail to provide such opportunities for students in their classes. In my experience in the schools, I have noted that teenagers, as well as teachers, quickly see through such hypocrisy. Nothing is more detrimental to the "teaching soul" of educators than knowing they are living a professional lie, knowing that their own school is failing to act on what they are teaching, preaching, and promising to students, or knowing that instead of lessons on how to improve their health, students are being offered lessons on how organizations such as schools use public-relations buzz words such as "leave no child behind" to gloss over program inadequacies and lack of staff commitment to the promised change process.

3. The wellness team model needs to include many outreach services that can quickly identify, intervene, educate, support, and refer students who are overweight, obese, or plagued by other health problems. Imagine students like Dylan, the young Bill Fibkins, and Naperville Central High School's Jennifer Mayor, Jessica Wolfrum, and Nadine Youssef surrounded by a variety of easily accessible intervention and education services.

4. The wellness team model needs to provide easy access to the school's nutrition and physical activity programs for healthy students so they continue to remain fit and offer healthy role models for their peers.

5. The wellness team model utilizes the school cafeteria and student dining experience as a laboratory to promote healthy eating choices for students and staff before school, during the school day, and after school hours. It should establish the cafeteria as an attractive place where students and staff want to congregate, share their dining experience as members of the school community, and in the process have easy access to information about developing a healthy lifestyle and, when needed, referrals

to school and community counseling, health, mental health, and recreation resources. As kitchen teacher Esther Cook of Martin Luther King Middle School in Berkeley, California, suggests, the school's dining experience should be enjoyable, even fun. She says, "It's very fun in here. It's really important to me that the students have fun."[3]

6. The wellness team model also requires outreach to the various curricula in the school, outreach that encourages teachers to provide information about nutrition and build physical activity into academic lessons. For example, teachers involved in the Physical Activity Across the Curriculum (PAAC) University of Kansas research project in the Kansas City and Topeka areas receive training and support, including myriad suggestions in a manual and on a website, for including physical activity in lessons about any subject: math, social studies, language arts, and science. While the PAAC model is focused on elementary school children, it does provide a model for secondary school wellness teams to consider in their effort to find creative new ways to increase information and physical activity in our large middle schools, junior high schools, and high schools.[4]

7. The wellness team model needs to offer easily accessible nutrition and physical activity programs for teaching staff, administrators, faculty, and support staff so they become and remain models for a healthy lifestyle, programs that offer early identification, education, and support when needed for the adults in the school who are responsible for caring for children.

8. The wellness team model needs to include an outreach to parents that offers easily accessible workshops on nutrition, participation in vigorous activity in the school and community recreation programs before and after school and work hours, such as the program led by Bill Carmichael in Hull, Massachusetts, and referrals and access to community health and mental health organizations. Simply put, parents have to be included in the school wellness model so they become partners with the schools in promoting physical activity and good

nutrition at home. Research from the federally funded Child and Adolescent Trial for Cardiovascular Health (CATCH) indicates that one of the reasons the project failed to reduce obesity in 5,000 third- through fifth-graders in ninety-six schools in four areas of the country was lack of family involvement.[5] Susan Okie suggests that CATCH was school centered and did not include a major effort to change what children did after school or at home. Leslie Lytle, a University of Minnesota epidemiologist, was a member of the research team that led the CATCH study. She told Okie, "While we could positively affect the school piece, kids' total calorie intake and energy expenditure is over a 24-hour period. The family is a huge piece of this. We're really struggling to get families engaged in all health promotions with kids."[6]

9. The wellness team also will need outreach to community recreation programs that can offer after-school opportunities for physical activity, education, mentoring supports, and referrals, similar to what I received from Bill Carmichael and the Hull recreation program. Schools can't be the only source of physical activity for students. If students leave school and lead a sedentary life without physical activity, the lessons learned in school about leading a healthy lifestyle will never take hold. Recreation personnel, like parents, can share in the effort and be important partners with the school, thereby offering a coordinated twenty-four-hour-a-day team effort.

10. Finally, the wellness team effort needs to embrace the latest technology to monitor important health indicators for students and staff and offer the same service to parents before and after school hours when possible, as part of the school's physical education and after-school recreation and education programs.

I call this model the Circle of Wellness because its goal is to provide ongoing attention to improving the health of every member of the school community. It's a whole-school approach that offers easy access for students, parents, and staff to intervention, education that encourages increased physical activity and healthier nutrition, mentoring, support, and referrals to school and community health and mental health and recreation services before school, during the school day, and after school hours. From my own work in education reform in the schools, I understand the harsh reality that implementing a Circle of Wellness will be filled with detours and barriers such as limited financial resources; educators who resist change and want to hang on to the "old PE" and who object to the schools' becoming major centers for health, nutrition, and physical activity; and administrators, teachers, parents, and community members who are conditioned to long-held rituals such as encouraging students to eat off campus, endorsing (particularly on the part of alumni) interscholastic sports competitions as the main component of the physical education program because athletic teams' participation can pay off in college scholarships and community pride; and viewing students' nutrition as an issue for families, not the school. As Naperville School Superintendent Donald Weber observes about the move to increase nutrition and physical activity for students, "It's an attitude adjustment. It's nice to have climbing walls and stuff we have in our school, but it's more about having students take responsibility for their fitness."[7]

A sea change is underway in the ways educators, students, parents, and community members view the opportunities for vigorous physical activity for *each* student in their schools. Awareness about the downside of traditional PE programs is increasing. For example, Bob Pangrazi, an Arizona State University physical education professor, says there is good evidence to change traditional PE even if you love team sports. Pangrazi points out that only 1% of all Americans play a team sport beyond age twenty-five, and the number is barely a fraction of that by the time people reach forty-five.[8] State and local legislators and educators are taking action. Reporter Bob Condor observes that the Texas legislature is considering a bill to require daily PE for students in kindergarten through sixth grade. Four Texas cities were cited in the ten top fattest cities, with Houston as number one.[9]

Condor also describes a successful effort spearheaded by a group of community members in Owensboro, Kentucky, to install fitness center equipment in six middle schools and one high school, complete with heart rate monitors. The cost was $50,000 to $75,000 per school, split evenly between the school district and the Owensboro Mercy Health System medical center. Debby Neel, a vice president at Owensboro Mercy, says, "We are called the barbecue capital of the world. We figured the health of the community might need some attention. We first started assessing students in 1996 and discovered 27 percent of fifth and sixth graders were overweight. We made it our mission to do something to reverse the pattern."[10]

Educators are learning that preaching and punishment to get teens to exercise don't work. New York City, the largest school district in the nation, has embarked on an ambitious plan to rebuild its physical education program. According to reporter Catherine A. Carroll, in 2004 the 1.1-million-student district had earmarked about $340 million to be spent over the next five years. Lori Benson, the district's director of fitness and physical education, said, "There is a childhood obesity crisis right here in the city." Ms. Benson said a 2003 study showed that 43% of elementary school children in the city were either overweight or obese. The new PE curriculum focuses on aerobic activity, flexibility, body composition and muscular strength, and an assessment, called a Fitnessgram, that provides parents with a fitness-level summary.[11]

The district has also started what Ms. Benson calls a "renaissance" middle school sports programs called CHAMPS, for Cooperative, Healthy, Active, Motivated, Positive Students. The program allows students to choose from a wide variety of after-school activities such as yoga or tai chi. The pilot program began in fifty middle schools in the spring of 2004 and as of November 2004 included one hundred schools, with 600 activities being offered.[12]

The Fitnessgram being used in New York City is becoming part of the "new PE" movement. Reporter John Gehring states that Darlene Groves was caught off guard when she received a physical fitness report from her daughter's school that ranked them in a "needs improvement" category and suggested they eat more vegetables and exercise more. The detailed update came from Fitzgerald Elementary School in Arlington, Texas, one of some 11,000 schools nationwide using the Fitnessgram to help make physical activity a part of students' daily life. In California lawmakers in 1996 required all students in the fifth, seventh, and ninth grades to be assessed by Fitnessgram.[13]

However, it is important to remind educators that fitness reports to parents need to be helpful, be hopeful, and provide clear, easily accessible avenues for intervention, education, and support. Simply put, while parents are used to receiving academic report cards, PE report cards are something new and may be unsettling if delivered without warning and with data that appear insensitive and intrusive. Reporter Bonnie Rothman Morris describes the reaction of parent Heather Jones when she got an unusual letter in the mail from the nurse at her son's school in Pennsylvania. The letter suggested that her nine-year-old son was too fat. Mrs. Jones was one of 400 parents in the 6,700 student East Penn school district to receive the same news. Mrs. Jones was not happy about the letter. "I took offense to it. I really thought it was inappropriate for the school to send a letter." The letter Mrs. Jones received regarding her eighty-five-pound son said the boy's body mass index indicated he was in the eighty-fifth percentile, putting him "at risk for overweight." Mrs. Jones argued that her son wasn't overweight at all. She said he towered over his classmates and was "just a big, healthy kid who's tall for his age."[14]

Rothman Morris says nationwide efforts to inform parents about weight and overall fitness of their children have met some resistance. Dr. William Dietz, director of the division of nutrition and physical activity at the Centers for Disease Control and Prevention, said the school letter Mrs. Jones received did call attention to the health risks of being overweight but failed to put the news in context and take the onus off the parents. Dietz says, "We're in the very early stage of recognition of overweight as a health problem. It's still widely perceived as a cosmetic issue."[15]

As the letter to parents in the East Penn school district suggests, there are stumbling blocks along the way in the battle to stem the epidemic of childhood and teen overweight and obesity. But I believe the good news far outweighs the setbacks and problems. Educators are learning the most effective ways to intervene to help kids and parents.

For example, Susan Okie describes the research of Tom Robinson, a Stanford University pediatrician, that suggests that people, especially kids, do things because they want to, not because someone has told them it's healthy. Robinson has learned the key lesson that the secret is to make people want to do things that are good for them. According to Okie, dance has become Robinson's stealth weapon in the battle to get kids to be more active: hip-hop, African dance, Mexican Ballet Folklorico, and Hawaiian hula. Instructors are teaching all of these styles to elementary and middle school girls as part of various studies Robinson and his team are conducting on obesity prevention.[16] Clearly, dance and movement can be included in many secondary school curricula, such as social studies, English, literature, science, math, language arts, business, and so forth.

Robinson's research to help stem the overweight and obesity epidemic is also breaking new ground with its multicomponent approach—encouraging children to exercise, trying to reduce the time they spend watching television or sitting at a computer, and teaching them to make healthier food choices. The Stanford Adolescent Heart-Health Program focused on tenth-graders in four ethnically diverse high schools and offered twenty lessons about diet, physical activity, and the health risks of smoking. It also taught teenagers specific skills about resisting peer pressure to smoke or adopt other unhealthy habits. Compared with students outside the program, tenth-graders in participating schools improved their diets, activity levels, and physical fitness and showed reductions in BMI and body fat.[17] It's an intervention program very similar to the Moorhead High School vignette described in chapter 1.

Change is taking place in the ways educators, community health, mental health and recreation professionals, and parents are acting to help children and teens make healthier food choices and become more physically active. The lessons being learned in this change process are that solutions are often simple and very doable when utilizing a community-wide intervention team of educators, parents, and community organizations. As Okie states, some of the most promising findings in preventing obesity suggest that an intervention model that is focused on getting children and teens to cut down on the amount of time being inactive along with engaging in increased physical activity, making healthier food choices, and receiving steady support and information about leading a healthier lifestyle can be very successful in helping overweight and obese teens lose weight.[18]

As reporter Amy Norton says, research in the *Archives of Pediatrics and Adolescent Medicine* suggests that children and teens may be more likely to exercise if they're motivated by fun and fitness rather than weight concerns. Norton describes a study of 200 students, with average ages of twelve and thirteen years, at one Pennsylvania middle school. Researchers found that "personal fulfillment" was the only motivation for being active.[19] That meant the kids tended to exercise for the sake of their health and athletic skills and to have fun, as Tom Robinson's research shows, and simply feel good, not in order to shed pounds or emulate their friends or parents.

The Circle of Wellness model I am proposing in this chapter is an effort to join and support the pioneering work of educators Ginny Reale and Phil Lawler, community leader Debby Neel, and school administrator Donald Weber and provide a whole-school approach that clearly spells out specific intervention services and how they are linked as a team to provide improved nutrition and physical activity for students, staff and parents. It is a model Debby Neel and other advocates for change can put forward as a plan to reverse the pattern of overweight, obesity, and other health problems, problems that in many cases limit academic achievement.

This model also takes into account the reality that 45.8 million people in the United States had no health insurance coverage in 2004 and 8.3 million of those were children, according to a U.S. Census report released in August 2003.[20] While schools should not be expected to bear full responsibility for keeping teens healthy, clearly school wellness teams can play an important role in prevention, education, early identification, support, and referral for students at risk of obesity, overweight, diabetes, cardiovascular disease, hypertension, and other problems.

The Circle of Wellness model I am proposing also embraces new uses of technology to aid in the effort to improve the health and well-being of students, parents, and staff. Many students, parents, and staff have personal computers, fax machines, and access to sending and receiving e-mails, telephone calls, and photos. The cost of a home PC continues to go down, and computers are becoming available to many families. For those families without a PC, these technical tools are available in many schools, public libraries, coffeehouses, and PC kiosks in the community. The result is that practically every student, educator, and parent has access to all the information, all the tools, and all the software to receive information from anyone in the world.

I argue that this technology breakthrough represents an asset we should take advantage of. As author Thomas L. Friedman suggests, "The Internet-e-mail-browser phase is all about me and my computer interacting with anyone, anywhere, on any machine, which is what e-mail is all about, and me and my computer interacting with anybody's website on the Internet, which is what browsing is all about. More people can now communicate and interact with more other people anywhere on the planet than ever before."[21] The communication Friedman is talking about can be used by schools to send and receive information electronically to and from individuals, groups, and the entire school community, including students, staff, and parents. That means information, education material, and monitoring results can be easily e-mailed to students, staff, and parents.

For example, let's focus on how parent-school communication can be improved in this technological age. Parent Heather Jones might have been more receptive to information about the possible health risks associated with her son's weight if she had access to a weekly online newsletter from the East Penn schools that asked for parent input and participation in a project to assess and monitor important health signs of students. Such a weekly online newsletter might include information about the newly mandated School Wellness Policy and programs being developed for students, staff, and parents like her. It would be a newsletter that invited an e-mail response and hopefully participation on her part before the weight notification program started and before the ill-fated letter was sent home.

This is just one example of how technology can increase participation and the flow of information among the whole school community. The new technology has the potential to replace the old
ways in which members of the school community interact. Educators no longer have to rely solely on such venues as school open
houses, PTA meetings, and teacher-parent conferences to engage in
dialogue with parents. Nor do parents have to show up physically at
these meetings to have access to information about their children's
progress in academics and fitness, especially those parents who are
already overburdened with work and family demands and
squeezed for time and those who have been turned off because of
conflicts with school personnel. The boundaries of communication
are no longer limited to an open house, a visit to school for a
teacher conference, and so forth. Communication can now take
place at any time and any place with schools joining the dot-org or
dot-edu movement.

An excellent example of the potential of the Internet and health
websites can be seen at Cleveland High School in Seattle, Washington. The University of Washington developed a Teen Smart website
at Cleveland. Carolyn Ahl and a group of nursing students and nurse
educators developed the site. As Ahl and her team suggest, the Internet is a daily presence in our lives and has created unprecedented
opportunities to transmit and share information, especially in the
domain of health education. Nurses and health-care providers are
now equipped with a powerful new tool for quickly reaching large
sectors of the population. Ahl points out that teenagers are one special population that is taking full advantage of the benefits the Internet has to offer. Adolescence is a crucial time in peoples' lives,
when they first begin to develop a strong sense of individuality as
they transition from childhood to adulthood. During this period lifelong patterns of problem-solving and health habits are developed.
Some teens develop health habits that are risky, such as poor nutritional habits, lack of physical exercise, tobacco use, alcohol and drug
use, and risky sexual behaviors. Ahl says that because most of these
risky health behaviors are preventable, providing high-risk teens
with information on health promotion is crucial. Today's teenagers'

medium of choice—the Internet—is the ideal vehicle for getting the word out in a format that is irresistible to young people.[22]

Those were the factors that prompted the University of Washington School of Nursing to explore the feasibility of developing a health-promotion Internet site that could be used to enhance health education in the high school classroom and provide a source of confidential information for students who are hesitant to identify and discuss personal health problems. The result was the Teen Smart website project, a community partnership with the faculty and students at Cleveland High School in Seattle's inner city. Cleveland High School serves a student body of 750 ethnically diverse and economically disadvantaged students.[23]

In the first stage of the project, the intervention team determined which health topics the students were most interested in. The main areas of interest and concern were related to weight, nutrition, drugs, sleep, and sex. Many students were reluctant to talk openly about sensitive areas of concern. The intervention team also determined that most students had high levels of access to computers and the Internet. All but 1% had used a computer, and 75% of the students said they used a computer at least once every week; 72% of the students had access to a computer at home, and 83% of those had access to the Internet. As Ahl suggests, this was a surprising finding given the high proportion of low-income and immigrant students in the school.[24]

To engage the students' interest and introduce them to the website's wide variety of information, the intervention team created special games and assignments tied in with each week's health education classroom context. Ahl says they were pleasantly surprised by the lack of difficulty the students experienced when completing assignments. The implementation of Teen Smart focused on raising the students' interest in health promotions (such as an online self-assessment quiz entitled "How Healthy Are You?") that were linked to topics covered in the weekly health education classes. The quizzes gave each student immediate individual feedback, scoring their health behaviors from low to high and providing them with links to other health-related websites relevant to their answers.[25]

Another Teen Smart feature, "Ask a Nurse," was designed to give students a private and confidential forum to discuss health questions with the Teen Health Center nurse practitioner. Individual students' questions were published and answered anonymously in the website's "Frequently Asked Questions" section so that all students could benefit from the information. The questions posed online were much more likely to address health concerns of a sensitive nature, such as sex and drugs, that they had been reluctant to volunteer publicly in focus groups.[26]

The "Discussion Board" was another Teen Smart feature. Supervised by the health education teachers, the board provided students with opportunities to analyze common life situations where decision-making is crucial to their health and safety. Each week the discussion board presented a problem-based scenario on health topics. Individual students could post a response describing what they would do in the situation and view other students' answers. The health education teachers were then able to use the posted responses for further class discussion.

Ahl and the intervention team measured the effectiveness of Teen Smart by including a feedback section in which students could click on and rate the website's features and assignments in areas such as ease of use, fun, usefulness, appropriateness, and relevance. The majority of the students, 78%, found Teen Smart to be interesting; 80% found it fairly easy to use; and 93% found it easy to understand. Asked to identify the most useful aspect of the project, the majority responded that the website contained health information they were interested in knowing about.[27]

The Teen Smart model appears to give students immediate, confidential access to information about the health issues they are grappling with, understanding of the health issues faced by peers, and opportunities to learn effective problem-solving skills to resolve problems and risky behavior, and it also aids educators in developing curricula that can better educate students, and themselves, on student health issues and using the counseling and referral resources of the nurse practitioner.

It appears that the Teen Smart model can provide school wellness teams with an immediate picture of student health concerns, identify additional intervention components that need to be provided for students in addition to health education and counseling by the nurse practitioner, and be able to move quickly to make these new intervention components available to students. As Mark Weber, spokesman for the Massachusetts Mental Health Services Administration, says, "Schools are stepping up to the plate and they've been very clever at helping students solve problems."[28]

Reporter Scott Allen provides a concrete example of the new thrust on the part of schools to lead the way in intervening to help students resolve health and personal issues. He cites data that school nurses now devote a third of their time to tending to children's health, emotional, and family issues rather than cuts and bruises only. Guidance counselors are spending half their time on health and mental health concerns rather than planning students' futures.[29] Change is occurring in the ways school nurses and guidance counselors have traditionally served students. Technology such as Teen Smart can be an important resource for nurses, guidance counselors, and school wellness teams by identifying what interventions students really need, not what educators and adults think they need.

The information schools can share is increasing at a fast pace. Schools nationwide weigh and measure students annually. They conduct vision, hearing, and scoliosis tests. However, as Dr. George Zioklowski, the director of pupil personnel services at the East Penn school district, points out, until recently most of this information "has been stuffed into a drawer."[30] Many school districts are beginning to add data about student health through programs such as Fitnessgram and the monitoring of important health signs, as in Naperville. A great deal of information about student health will also be available as local wellness policies are implemented. Technology tools are readily available right now in most schools to raise student, staff, and parent awareness about health, nutrition, and physical activity; monitor important student health signs such as blood pressure, cholesterol, and blood sugar levels; and develop regular fitness report cards for students and a fitness profile and report for the school, identifying how students are progressing. If we are going to integrate student health and physical activity into our curricula, they need to be measured just as academic progress is. Measurable data will be needed by school wellness teams to convince administrators, staff, parents, taxpayers, and even students that the team's Circle of Wellness plan is working to improve students' health and is a re- source to identify negative trends that need early intervention.

For example, what does the data developed by PE teachers Marge Edgar and Tony Jankowski, school nurse Barbara Grant, student as- sistance counselor Brad Langdon, and dietitian Nancy Clifford tell administrator Al Morris, staff, students, parents, community mem- bers, and health, mental health, and recreation resources about the overall health of Moorhead's ninth through twelfth grade students? Are there differences between grade levels? What interventions seem to work best for different groups, such as males, females, or specific grades?

And which wellness interventions seem to work best with staff? Are they seeing gains in their health due to participation in the wellness team programs? What interventions work best to address the con- cerns of parents about their children's health and that of themselves and other family members? What are the observations of community health, mental health, and recreation professionals? Do they observe an improvement in the health and well-being of students? These ques- tions are examples of how data gathering can help to keep school well- ness teams on the path that offers the biggest health payoff for the food service, physical education, nursing, counseling, health educa- tion, after-school recreation, and parent support budgets.

In addition to clear strategies and knowledge of new physical ed- ucation and nutrition programs that are being developed in schools, a successful Circle of Wellness model requires the identification of specific components within the circle that offer many open doors of help for overweight, obese, and unhealthy students like Dylan and healthy students who need daily opportunities to stay healthy. These components represent the nuts and bolts of the whole-school approach to promoting a healthy lifestyle model for students.

In a sense these components give the wellness team's efforts a very strong and positive identity within the school organization. While I have identified many of these components in previous chapters, I believe it is helpful to the reader to summarize and further elaborate on these open doors for help.

- A school dining experience that offers healthy food in an attractive setting and offers information on health, diet, and nutrition and referrals to school and community counseling, health, mental health, and recreation resources
- A before-school breakfast program for students and staff that includes opportunities to begin the day with a healthy breakfast and connect socially with other members of the school community
- Dietitians who offer workshops for students, staff, and parents on healthy food preparation and diet
- Vending machines that offer healthy food and drink options as well as easily accessible water
- School nurses who provide health counseling; team with PE teachers to monitor health indicators such as weight, blood pressure, cholesterol, and blood sugar levels; participate in collecting Fitnessgram data; lead a forty-eight-hour support program to help students maintain a healthy lifestyle on weekends; team with faculty to integrate health and physical activity lessons into the various curricula; provide student, parent, and staff referrals to community agencies; and offer outreach to staff and parents
- Student assistance counselors who offer individual and group counseling to students, train peer counselors, lead parent support groups, team with faculty to integrate health and physical activity lessons into various curricula, participate in collecting Fitnessgram data, and provide referrals to community agencies and outreach to staff and parents
- Physical education teachers who provide daily opportunities for vigorous physical activity for students, team with the school nurse to monitor important health indicators of students, team

with faculty to integrate health and physical activity lessons into curricula, participate in collecting Fitnessgram data, utilize the resources of community health professionals, such as Naperville's Dr. Bufalino, in the new PE program, and provide students and parents with referrals when needed

- Teacher advisors who offer support and referral opportunities to students and parents and serve on the front lines as early detectors of unhealthy student behaviors
- Administrators who lead the effort to prepare a Fitnessgram to be sent home semiannually to parents of each student; an online newsletter that describes wellness team activities and provides information on health, nutrition, and physical activity and the availability of community resources; and coordination with community health, mental health, and recreation agencies
- A Child Study Team (CST) that encourages student referrals from administrators, teachers, and support staff for health as well as academic problems
- After-school recreation programs that are fun; give teenagers a positive after-school option; and offer the opportunity for physical activity, tutoring, healthy snacks and drinks, and participation in healthier cookery clubs and growing clubs, activities that can also include staff and parents
- A staff wellness program that offers opportunities for physical activity, monitoring of important health signs, workshops on health and nutrition, and referrals to community health, mental health, and recreation agencies
- When possible, an evening parent wellness program offered in collaboration with community health, mental health, and recreation agencies and featuring opportunities for physical activity, monitoring of important health signs, workshops on health and nutrition, and referrals when needed

This whole-school approach has the potential to guide overweight, obese, and unhealthy students into health-promoting activities throughout the day and evening, offering many open doors throughout the day that students can walk through and learn about how to develop and maintain a healthy lifestyle. It also offers staff members the opportunity to collaborate with each other in an important mission to help unhealthy students, not remain isolated, and improve their own health and well-being.

As researchers Floretta Dukes McKenzie and Julius B. Richmond suggest, because most schools do not have cohesive policies for enhancing healthy student development, most school health programs are developed in relative isolation. In general the tendency is to rely on narrowly focused, short-term, cost-intensive interventions that serve a small proportion of students in a noncomprehensive way.[31]

In contrast, my whole-school approach targets the health and well-being of each and every student in the school. That is, it provides for intervention for unhealthy students as well as health promotion for healthy students. It does not use the school's intervention and prevention resources and efforts on a small percentage of students who may be acting out, potential dropouts, suicidal, or involved in substance abuse. Promoting opportunities to develop a healthy lifestyle can help redirect these marginal students to become contributing members of the school community, inviting them into attractive and fun doors offered in the school's Circle of Wellness, a circle that can envelop a student with care, guidance, hope, and the opportunity to change unhealthy habits.

NOTES

1. Susan Okie, *Fed Up! Winning the War Against Childhood Obesity* (Washington, DC: Joseph Henry Press, 2005), 188.

2. Okie, *Fed Up!* 207.

3. Okie, *Fed Up!* 185.

4. Okie, *Fed Up!* 113–17.

5. Okie, *Fed Up!* 205–7.

6. Okie, *Fed Up!* 205–7.

7. Linda Yu, "Learner for Life: 'New PE,'" ABC.com, 3 Dec. 2003, http://abclocal.go.com/wls/news/specialsegments_Nov02/020903_ss_Learner.html (accessed 27 June 2005).

8. Bob Condor, "Playing Games With PE: With Kids' Health in Mind, a Few Bright Spots Buck the Trend to an End of Gym Classes," *Chicago Tribune*, 10 Mar. 2002, http://www.pe4life.org/playinggamesspe.php (accessed 27 June 2005).

9. Condor, "Playing Games."

10. Condor, "Playing Games."

11. Catherine A. Carroll, "N.Y.C. Renews Physical Education Efforts," *Education Week*, 24 Nov. 2004, http://www.edweek.org/ew/articles/2004/11/24/13physed.h24.html (accessed 25 May 2005).

12. Carroll, "N.Y.C. Renews Physical Education Efforts."

13. John Gehring, "Fitness Report Cards Part of 'New PE' Movement," *Education Week*, 19 June 2002, http://www.edweek.org/ew/articles/2002/06/19/41gym.h21.html? (accessed 25 June 2005).

14. Bonnie Rothman Morris, "Letters on Students' Weight Ruffle Parents," *New York Times*, 26 Mar. 2002, F7.

15. Rothman Morris, "Letters on Students' Weight," F7.

16. Okie, *Fed Up!* 128, 129.

17. Okie, *Fed Up!* 128, 129.

18. Okie, *Fed Up!* 128, 129.

19. Amy Norton, "Kids Exercise to Feel Good, Not Lose Weight," Reuters, 8 Dec. 2005, http://news.yahoo.com/s/nm/20051208/hl_nm/kids_weight_dc_1 (accessed 21 Dec. 2005).

20. Alan Eisner, "Mobile Clinic Tries to Fill Health Needs," Reuters, 30 Dec. 2005, http://news.yahoo.com/s/nm/20051230/ts_nm/life_clinicdc (accessed 31 Dec. 2005).

21. Thomas L. Friedman, *The World Is Flat* (New York: Farrar, Straus and Giroux, 2005), 71.

22. Carolyn Ahl, "Helping At-Risk Kids Get 'Teen Smart,'" minority nurse.com, 27 Jan. 2002, http://www.minoritynurse.com/features/undergraduate/01-27-02g.html (accessed 10 May 2004). Originally published in *Minority Nurse* magazine (Winter 2002).

23. Ahl, "Helping At-Risk Kids."

24. Ahl, "Helping At-Risk Kids."

25. Ahl, "Helping At-Risk Kids."

26. Ahl, "Helping At-Risk Kids."

27. Ahl, "Helping At-Risk Kids."

28. Scott Allen, "Schools Shoulder Load for Mental Health Care," boston.com, 29 Dec. 2005, http://www.boston.com/yourlife/health/mental/articles/2005/12/29/schools_shoulder_load (accessed 29 Dec. 2005).

29. Allen, "Schools Shoulder Load."

30. Rothman Morris, "Letters on Students' Weight," F7.

31. Floretta Dukes McKenzie and Julius B. Richmond, "Linking Health and Learning: An Overview of Coordinated School Health Programs," in *Health Is Academic*, ed. Eva Marx and Susan Frelick Wooley (New York: Teachers College Press, 1998), 8–9.

7

UTILIZING THE CIRCLE OF WELLNESS TO ADDRESS STAFF OVERWEIGHT, OBESITY, AND RELATED HEALTH PROBLEMS

I argue that the Circle of Wellness also needs to include opportunities for administrators, faculty, and support staff to learn about how to develop and maintain a healthy lifestyle and be health role models for their peers, students, parents, and citizen taxpayers. What is most surprising and in fact detrimental to developing a healthy school environment is that the health and well-being of staff members is often given a low priority or left out of the intervention plan. Staff wellness seems to be an afterthought and is given little support and resources. Yet these are the staff members who administer; teach; counsel; prepare food; monitor cafeterias, school grounds, and athletic and musical events; serve as secretaries, custodians, and bus drivers; and interact daily with students.

In many schools these important caregivers and role models are left on their own to develop personal efforts to stay healthy, a process that works for some, mainly those who are younger and more active, but leaves many others without the necessary intervention as they age. Students observe these caregivers, note their health and well-being, and notice when they are overweight, obese, or in poor health. They take notice when teachers have high absentee rates, lack energy to complete necessary tasks, and lash out at students for no apparent reason. They notice when an obese school secretary is ill-tempered and constantly munching on doughnuts and sweets and when overweight school grounds monitors ask students to bring back a lunch from a fast-food restaurant. They notice when staff members openly talk abut an overweight and overworked administrator "heading for a heart attack if he keeps up his crazy pace and doesn't lose some weight." Kids listen to what adults say to each other in school families as well as in their own families, and sometimes whispers are early warnings of trouble to come.

For staff, "personal efforts" to change unhealthy eating, drinking, and behavior habits often begin with a New Year's resolution, a bad report from a visit to a doctor, or the serious illness of a family member or coworker that sends a wake-up call. The message might be, "Hey, Joe was only forty-three. The kids in his classes loved him. What a loss! If only he had watched his weight and listened to the concerns of his wife, kids, and colleagues, he would be here today. I tried to help him, but he always said, 'Hey, don't worry about me. I am starting a new diet and exercise workout tomorrow. I promise!'" But good intentions and promises, as we all know, are often not enough and gradually slip away. As readers know from their own life experiences, resolutions built on "personal efforts" usually falter without intervention, education, monitoring, and support.

The lack of programs to bring attention to the importance of staff wellness can be seen in local wellness policies. For example, the National Alliance for Nutrition and Activity (NANA) "Model Local School Wellness Policies on Physical Activity and Nutrition" does state that school districts need to "plan and implement activities and policies that support personal efforts by staff to maintain a healthy lifestyle."[1] But there is no identification of possible activities, information on how and when they would be offered, or explanation of why the emphasis on staff wellness is limited to only "personal efforts." In the NANA model there is no attention to the responsibility school districts have to provide health intervention for administrators, faculty, and support staff so they are fit to do their work with optimum energy and motivation and can deliver quality instruction, care, and support to students each day.

The Model Wellness Policy Guide developed by the Center for Ecoliteracy does not even give staff wellness a priority. There is a section on "professional development" that calls for "regular professional development at least annually to teachers and the Food Service staff on basic nutrition, nutritional education and benefits of sustainable agriculture."[2] Important training it is, but again, there is no mention of intervention and education to promote staff health and well-being and the role of staff as models of healthy lifestyles for students, parents, and taxpayers.

I don't believe the NANA and Center for Ecoliteracy wellness models knowingly give little attention to the importance of staff intervention in local wellness policies. The issues involved in overweight and obesity in schools are focused on students. Staff wellness is not on the radar screen of many educators, activists, and researchers. Wellness for staff has traditionally been given a low intervention priority even though, as I have observed in my work and research, there are staff members who are clearly overweight, obese, and in poor health. Everyone in the school community seems to know about overweight, obese, and unhealthy staff members. Gossip that includes negative labeling about staff who are struggling with health issues travels fast in schools, and the labeling is often very hostile, similar to the name-calling of overweight and obese students.

However, in addition to the gossip and negative labeling, there are leaders in the schools who are searching for ways to intervene and help unhealthy workers. In my conversations with school nurses I have listened to their concerns about staff members who are overweight and obese and have elevated blood pressure, cholesterol, and blood sugar levels, concerns that these staff members are at risk of serious health problems and are ignoring the flashing red light of danger ahead. I have listened to concerns from administrators, department heads, teachers, and civil service workers who observe fellow workers headed on a downward health cycle. Adults in the school know when colleagues are at risk of health problems, just as students know with their peers.

The symptoms that accompany being unhealthy are very notice-able in most cases. They show. Yet concerned union leaders, admin-istrators, and colleagues are often hesitant to intervene because they can't offer remedies except to suggest "personal efforts." Adminis-trators are reluctant to tie overweight and obesity problems to poor workplace performance, a charge they feel will be strongly opposed by the teacher unions, civil service unions, some members of the faculty and student body, and parents. However, in my experience this practice of looking the other way gives no comfort to adminis-trators and fellow workers who daily observe a peer struggling to be effective, not having others notice their dilemma, and making a "personal effort" to change that isn't paying off.

I believe implementing a staff-centered intervention plan as part of a Circle of Wellness has the potential to address the concerns of fellow workers who want to help and offers overweight, obese, and unhealthy staff many open doors to change unhealthy habits. The Circle of Wellness interventions also offer healthy staff ongoing health-promotion activities and the opportunity to be healthy role models for their peers. The Circle of Wellness can help break down the professional and personal distance and isolation between ad-ministrators, faculty, and support staff. It can be a humanizing ex-perience in which each person, like each student, can hopefully be-gin to assume responsibility for his or her own health with intervention, education, support, and, when needed, referrals to community health, mental health, and recreation agencies. The Cir-cle of Wellness offers students and staff a "we are all in this to-gether" option to improve health, an option that can help to prevent diseases and reduce the risk of poor health for both high-risk and low-risk staff and students; reduce medical expenses for staff, stu-dents, and their families; reduce absenteeism and poor work perfor-mance by staff as well as absenteeism and poor academic perfor-mance by students; and offer health promotion, education, and support for parents.

The staff component in the Circle of Wellness shines a needed light on the negative impact that overweight, obesity, and related health problems can have on the staff affected and the drag that these health problems can have on the school's ability to be a successful organization in which each employee is ready and set to deliver an excellent education to students. I offer the following examples of employee wellness model programs utilized in the business sector and in some state governments, models that school wellness teams can consider in their efforts to make staff wellness a reality in their schools. These program models are also food for thought, meant to stimulate alternative ways of thinking about possibilities by wellness team members and to raise the question, If wellness programs for employees are so important in companies such as State Farm and DaimlerChrysler and in state governments such as Arkansas, why are wellness efforts for employees at all levels either nonexistent or a rarity in our nation's schools?

- The State Farm program: According to an American Diabetes Association case study, State Farm offers its more than 72,000 employees across the country an array of helpful health programs and activities focusing on prevention and education. Voluntary, free health exams are the cornerstone of its health promotion efforts and are offered to every employee at ages twenty-five, thirty, and thirty-five; every other year from forty to fifty, and annually after fifty. These thorough exams held on-site provide employees with opportunities to catch health issues early and to manage their own health proactively. Periodic, popular walking challenges encourage State Farm employees to incorporate walking into their workday. At any given time during the workday, walking groups can be seen getting their steps. Yoga, Pilates, and Weight Watchers at Work classes are held on an ongoing basis for State Farm headquarters employees, and many offices have on-site fitness programs such as walking or running clubs and Pilates and Jazzercise classes. State Farm also offers national discounts to Bally Total Fitness clubs and Gold's Gym. To help in weight management, State Farm has worked with cafeteria vendors to provide healthy eating choices. State Farm also sponsors health fairs and "Lunch and Learn" seminars to provide a variety of educational opportunities for employees. Individual State Farm offices select specific health topics that are of interest to their employees, including obesity, physical activity, and eating right. "Lunch and Learn" is also available online as part of the company's Internet classes. In addition, for decades the State Farm Park has offered Bloomington, Illinois–area employees and their families a wonderful opportunity to be physically outdoors by swimming, playing tennis and basketball, and so forth.[3] From a school perspective, it is interesting that part of State Farm's mission is to help customers "manage the risks of everyday life." It appears that State Farm also works hard to do this for employees through its "intensive, ongoing efforts to help them recognize that healthy behavior such as eating right and getting regular physical activity are critical to disease prevention and management, and by offering an environment in which to pursue these critical activities."[4] It sounds like a good slogan, platform, and identity for school wellness teams, helping students, parents, and staff to "manage the risks of everyday life."

- The United Auto Workers (UAW) Health and Fitness Programs: Steve Cherniak, human resource associate for Ford Motor Company, indicates,

We have 56 UAW-Ford fitness centers around the country. All but one are in manufacturing locations. All UAW-Ford fitness centers are equipped with cardiovascular and strength equipment. Through the years we've had as high as 50% of the eligible population enrolled at one time or another. We are getting our people to be more physically active at all ages and at all stages of their lives because the health benefits of physical activity are enormous. Physical activity should absolutely be part of disease prevention and management. Fitness centers have the greatest impact of keeping low risk employees at low risk. The core of employees that you will first accommodate are those who exercise anyway, but you are giving them a much more convenient place to do it. We want to continue to give them a reason not to stop their exercising routine.[5]

This sounds to me like another excellent slogan, platform, and identity for school wellness teams: fitness and health intervention in order to keep employees with low health risk at low risk.

- The Coca-Cola Company/Singapore Ministry of Health Staff "Step With It Singapore" program: On May 19, 2004, as part of a continuing effort to promote a more active and healthy lifestyle among its staff, the Ministry of Health (MOH) announced it was introducing the first workplace "Step With It Singapore" program. The announcement also indicated that MOH will launch an internal health database and website for staff. The site monitors individual health status and rewards each staff member with points for participating in healthy lifestyle activities. The database includes employees' personal health profile and results of annuals health screening or any other health checks conducted by their own specialists or through monthly lunchtime sessions at MOH. MOH is the first workplace in Singapore to implement the "Step With It Singapore" program. All 400 staff members were given a personal stepometer, a device that monitors the number of steps a person takes, to track their step count over a twelve-month period. To encourage staff to achieve and exceed the daily target of 10,000 steps, the MOH Health Promotion Committee (HPC) introduced several lifestyle initiatives, which include increasing the frequency of activities with high-impact exercises; starting a variety of sports clubs with regular weekly activities such as jogging, bowling, badminton, table tennis, and so forth; organizing inter-divisional and inter-institutional sporting events; and participating in external sports events such as the Singapore Marathon. Staff are able to track their daily steps by keying the data into the new web-based database system. Incentives in the form of rewards and prizes will be awarded to staff who achieve the target or highest number of steps over designated periods. Divisions whose staff attain the highest total of steps will also be awarded prizes. The "Step With It" program was also launched with 30,000 teachers and students in twelve schools and extends its reach to adult in the workplace starting with MOH. "Step With It" was first introduced in the

United States by the Coca-Cola Company in 2002, with the objective being to engage students in physical activity, and was tested in April 2002 in middle schools in Houston, Philadelphia, and Atlanta. The program was supported by the National Association of Sports and Physical Education. In the Singapore pilot, 76% of students made an extra effort to increase their daily counts. The program was associated with fun and feeling energetic and healthy. The program was expected to reach 5,000 working adults in Singapore by the end of 2004.[6] "Step With It" could also be another slogan and platform and could help create an identity for school wellness teams. Imagine inter-institutional competition with "Step With It" and sports events among teams from the English, social studies, science, math, language arts, physical education and health, technology, business, and pupil personnel services departments and the administration and support staff! How about competitions among jogging, bowling, badminton, basketball, softball, swimming, table tennis, and other clubs? These activities could generate new energy to promote physical activity among adults in the schools. And how about starting a parent "Step With It" program and sports clubs? Imagine a web-based database health system in which employees can view and update their own health-related details and that offers medical checkups at monthly lunchtime sessions, as is done at MOH.

- The Pitney-Bowes Obesity Initiative: J. Brent Pawlecki, MD, associate medical director for Pitney-Bowes, says the company, particularly with its aging workforce, has not escaped the epidemic of obesity in the United States. The company's medical expenses directly attributed to obesity were estimated at $5.6 million in 2002. Obesity is likely to be a significant indirect factor in Pitney-Bowes's medical expenses for both fully insured and self-insured employees. The reality is that preventing obesity is considerably cheaper than treating people once they become obese. Obesity and other health-related problems must be addressed in the company's successful wellness initiatives and as a business imperative, focusing on how the epidemic affects the company. Pawlecki identifies the following strategies to address the obesity issue at Pitney-Bowes: the creation of a "WebMD" tool to expand personal health information access via the Internet; preventive services such as cardiovascular and diabetes screening; behavioral health and disease management programs; weight loss, fitness, and nutrition education included in wellness initiatives; a registered dietitian serving as a valuable team member in the medical and wellness programs; health professionals offering teaching and counseling in the seven on-site medical clinics; a dietitian to work with local food services to provide regular healthy choice options; numerous health and fitness seminars; Weight Watchers programs available at work-site locations; fitness centers provided at some work-site locations; and activity and exercise fitness programs such as walking programs provided through work-site initiatives. Along with these proposed strategies, Pawlecki describes a "Supportive Corporation," which includes senior management tackling health and obesity problems as a business priority; transforming the internal corporate culture to include health and fitness awareness, which will increase employee effectiveness and productivity and control some of the rising health costs; using "inspirational power talks" to address employee health; encouraging participation of top leadership in fitness and wellness activities, serving as examples for other employees; prominently featuring health and obesity tools on the WebMD site; increasing prominence of "Health and Well-Being News" on the Pitney-Bowes Internet home page; minimizing conflicting messages about health, such as promoting exercise but at the same time increasing fitness center dues; increasing Pitney-Bowes Internet access for the highly diverse Pitney-Bowes workforce; maximizing the use of health education seminars and counseling services made available by health professionals in the seven on-site medical clinics; having vending machines that make nutritional food and drink available; promoting bottled water and healthy food and drink at company meetings; promoting walking trails and clubs at company sites; launching a corporate "Know Your BMI" campaign through wellness initiatives; implementing a discount program for fitness center membership; and implementing through corporate procurement a single nationwide vending machine contract mandating healthier choices with variable pricing based on nutritional content. Pawlecki reports, "The initial evaluation of the WebMD Health Risk Appraisal completed by Pitney-Bowes employees reveals that 80% of people have poor diet and 85% are not within their normal weight range. Additionally, 61% are physically inactive. These scores are higher than for the general population."[7] I believe the Pitney-Bowes intervention plan includes many components that school wellness teams need to consider as they put together a Circle of Wellness model that fits their school. For example, imagine a WebMD Internet site that employees could access daily, a site that contains health information; dates, times, and locations of Circle of Wellness activities in the school; and notices about health activities and resources in the community. One click and school employees would be connected to health options. In fact, "One click can get you connected to better health" could be a powerful slogan and platform and could help create an identity for the school wellness team.

- The DaimlerChrysler Corporate Wellness Program: Health reporter Jennifer Hutchins says that Gordon Ondrisek is a "Stay-Well Groupie." The senior engineer at DaimlerChrysler headquarters in Auburn Hills, Michigan, regularly attends Stay-Well seminars, watches health videos from the on-site library, and even acts as a Stay-Well delegate to spread the word on wellness among his coworkers. The DaimlerChrysler wellness program is a three-way collaboration with the United Auto Workers (UAW) and Stay-Well, an international provider of health management services, and reaches 81,000 employees at twenty-six locations nationwide. Representative from each body form a Wellness Advisory Committee that holds on-site meetings to discuss the best approach for each location. "At every location we identify top risks," says Mary Kaufman, Stay-Well's senior program manager for DaimlerChrysler. The program has endured for fifteen years even though there have been many changes at Chrysler and includes employee health appraisals with voluntary questionnaires and blood screening to assess such factors as stress, diet, fitness, blood pressure, and cholesterol levels. An online health risk appraisal is also available. Hutchins reports that if a site has large numbers of employees with high blood pressure, for example, Stay-Well implements educational programs to help diminish that problem. At every location, professional educators deliver seminars and workshops on topics that range from fitness to disease prevention. On average, two seminars are held each month. Site-wide campaigns also help employees to jump-start their healthy lifestyles. During a campaign employees might track their liquid intake or how many servings of vegetables they eat each day. Participants earn "WellBucks," which they can redeem for health-related items such as pedometers. Hutchins suggests that while the wellness programs are designed to be fun, the objectives are serious. Individuals who are at risk in two or more health categories are eligible for the NextStep program, which involves telephone counseling from Stay-Well experts. Mary Kaufman says, "If you are at risk for nutrition, you would be hooked up with a registered dietician. It's totally voluntary and totally confidential as well." Walter Horton, a business analyst, says the wellness initiatives have helped him to make health a top priority. He enjoys taking a break from the workday to attend seminars and is dedicated to eating well and working out at the on-site fitness center. "I benefit from some of the things in the program." Dr. David Anderson, vice-president of the Stay-Well Company, says awareness, assessment, education, and maintenance are the building blocks of the Stay-Well program.[8] While school wellness teams don't have a connection with the Stay-Well program, clearly the pitch to employees that includes the slogan "Stay Well Through Awareness, Assessment, Education and Maintenance (AAEM)" can help create a powerful platform and identity for the wellness team.

- The Healthy Arkansas Initiative: Reporter Gina Bellafante suggests that Governor Mike Huckabee's own weight loss and health transformation led him to begin the Healthy Arkansas Initiative in the spring of 2004. The goal of the program is to persuade men, women, and children statewide to join him in his new embrace of healthy eating, drinking, and physical exertion. Under the program all state employees are now given thirty minutes a day to exercise. Another incentive offered is a point system that allows those working for the state to accrue days off when they lose weight, stop smoking, or exhibit other signs of sound body stewardship. Huckabee gives the following example of a reward system that is out of whack. "Someone calls in sick and you say, 'Are you sick?' They answer, 'Well, I'm 50 pounds overweight and don't get off my rear and I am sick.'" Huckabee says that kind of day-off reward is ridiculous. "You get rewarded for being sick and the poor guy who is slogging away exercising gets to work." It sounds familiar, doesn't it? Unhealthy school employees call in sick and get the day off, and healthy workers have to show up.[9] It's a scenario in which worker absenteeism is allowed to flourish while health problems go unaddressed in most schools. As Huckabee suggests, how about an intervention plan that rewards employees for being healthy and productive and having a low absentee rate? How about an intervention plan that addresses the fifty-pounds-overweight guy or gal who is unhealthy and unproductive and has a high absentee rate? His or her classes are regularly taught by a substitute, often with no lesson plans or previous contact with students. Or, in the case of support staff such as a bus driver, the job is done by a substitute who barely knows the route. It all adds up to wasted days for the unhealthy employee, for the students, and for administrators who have to provide coverage for employees who are regulars on the sick list. How about the school wellness team considering some of Huckabee's suggestions, such as thirty minutes to exercise and time off or other rewards for good attendance, stopping smoking, losing weight? Perhaps school wellness teams should also borrow some of Huckabee's reality-based approach to the health of employees by considering ideas such as "Being here counts. What you have to offer will be missed if you are ill. Let us help you get and stay healthy."

Again I raise the question, why aren't more schools developing similar wellness programs? Clearly, education leaders may be hesitant because they fear added cost to taxpayers, are concerned they can't successfully market the program to taxpayers and employees, and, probably most important, fail to see the link between employee wellness and reductions in absenteeism and health costs and increased productivity. Here is an argument and supporting data they can use to increase their own awareness about employee wellness programs and to sell staff, parents, and taxpayers on the need for such a program.

Let's begin with cost. Research by Erfurt, Footem, and Henirck estimate that a comprehensive work-site wellness program costs an employer between $70 and $130 per employee annually and that even the simplest of these programs have demonstrated a reduction in health-care costs, inpatient stays, and sick leave.[10] Health reporter Malin Lundblad says the cost of a corporate wellness program averages about $200 per employee each year.[11] What is the rationale for a school wellness program? First of all, using the above data one can see that these are manageable costs given the potential returns in improved employee health, lower absenteeism rates, lower turnover, and heightened morale and productivity.

As human resources expert Stephanie Sullivan Pittman, PHR, suggests, employee wellness programs have long been advocated as a way to maintain and improve employee health, reduce health care, reduce absenteeism, and increase productivity. Sullivan Pittman says several researchers have studied the impact of exercise on job performance. For example, NASA found that while the productivity of nonexercising office workers decreased 50% during the final two hours of the workday, the exercisers worked at full efficiency all day. Sullivan Pittman also says that several industry studies have demonstrated reductions in absenteeism and disability time as a result of employee wellness programs.[12]

While studies at DuPont and General Mills found 14–19% reductions, General Electric reported an astounding 45% decrease in absenteeism. Sullivan Pittman points out that wellness programs have the added benefit of recruiting and retaining high-achieving employees.[13] Employee wellness programs can contribute to a reduction in cardiac risks. Research by Heirich and Associates found a 35–45% reduction in overall cardiac risk among participants in a physical fitness program over a three-year period.[14] Research by Larry Chapman also found strong evidence that wellness programs that target hypertension control, physical activity, nutrition, and tobacco use were effective in altering employee behavior. Programs that targeted hypertension were found to have the greatest impact on health-care costs.[15]

Sullivan Pittman says programs that have shown the greatest return on investment have included the following major components: assessment activities that determine employee health and are used to identify health risks and provide insight to employers as to what the most pressing health issues are in their organizations; health screening for early detection and treatment of health problems; communication material such as newsletters, paycheck stuffers, posters, and bulletin board notices distributed or posted on an ongoing basis to provide accurate wellness updates; self-help materials; availability of self-care programs such as workshops, nurse advice lines, self-care software, and educational and promotional material on self-care; the use of incentives to reward people for healthy behavior; and involving the employee's family in the wellness program.[16]

Sullivan Pittman stresses the value of self-care in wellness program health promotions. She says studies show that about 75% of people who receive a self-care guide will use it at least one time within six months. Of all the items included in implementing a wellness program, the inclusion of self-care appears to provide the most consistent return on investment. She also warns that leaving spouses and dependents out of wellness programs may be unwise, as they account for 70% of all health care costs. She says that only 30% of wellness programs reviewed offered participation to spouses and dependents.[17]

How about a low-cost wellness model for schools? Sullivan Pittman advises, and she might well be talking to school administrators and wellness team leaders, "Programs do not necessarily have to be as extensive as those of the large corporations in order to have impact on employee health."[18] She suggests that smaller organizations can make inexpensive changes in the work environment such as offering health food in the cafeteria and vending machines, inviting the Red Cross, the American Heart Association, the American Cancer Society, and other organizations to conduct education workshops at the company's facility, offering flex-time for employees who want to exercise at lunchtime, providing showers and locker room facilities at work sites, providing information to employees by distributing free brochures and wellness newsletters, adding bike racks to the parking area, providing free health screenings, encouraging employee access to free electronic health newsletters, and providing partial reimbursement for membership to off-site health and exercise facilities.[19]

Sullivan Pittman's list of inexpensive changes in the work environment is very doable. We are not talking a spa experience here with mud bath, massages, and MRIs. This is a no-frills wellness model. I believe school wellness teams can utilize these components as building blocks in making local wellness policies a reality. More Circle of Wellness components can be added as the program evolves. Clearly there are strong, supportive data to suggest that a school wellness intervention for employees contributes to decreased absenteeism, reduced staff turnover, and improvement in the ability of employees to perform their jobs and provides an incentive to attract and retain highly achieving employees. School wellness teams need to keep in mind a report by the Radical HealthWorks organization that says that workers spend 30–50% of their waking hours at work; that food eaten at work contributes significantly to the total day's intake; that most employees will eat at work nearly every day, allowing for regular nutrition education in the workplace cafeteria or break room; that workplace social networks already exist that can be beneficial for encouraging and supporting healthy lifestyle habits; and, as First Chicago Corporation found in a survey of 3,066 of their employees, that as employees' BMI increases, the number of sick days, medical claims, and health-care costs go up.[20]

Speaking of taxpayers, at one point in my career I was developing a student assistance counseling program in a suburban high school. The school district included a large senior citizen condominium complex. Each year the residents of the condo village would turn out in droves to vote against the school budget. However, as part of the school wellness effort the district invited local citizens to use the school's weight rooms and fitness facilities before school, after school, and in the evening. Guess what? Many senior citizens flocked to the facilities and became pro-school and "yes" voters at budget time. They found a needed health resource and got to know other community members (senior citizens can be very isolated in "condo-land"), school employees, parents, and, most important, students who used the facilities. This wellness promotion brought together diverse members of the community in a positive way.

In conclusion, my Circle of Wellness is an inclusion model that can offer unhealthy and healthy students, parents, and staff concrete ways to improve and maintain a healthy lifestyle. This healthy lifestyle can help them to be better prepared to handle the career and personal issues they will surely face and avoid the health problems that can sap their will, energy, and hope as well as their financial resources. Schools are ideally situated to deliver such health interventions by reconfiguring their personnel and resources and, as Sullivan Pittman suggests, providing inexpensive interventions. Such interventions can benefit the health and well-being of every member of the school community. Local wellness policies may well be the vehicle that is needed to implement school wellness programs.

Clearly wellness policies are desperately needed to improve the health of children, teens, educators, and parents. There are *things* educators can do and *actions* they can take. For example, as writer Henry Fountain says, a disease like diabetes gallops practically out of control, with estimates that 21 million Americans have it and 45 million could develop it, yet relatively few people worry about it or alter their behavior to postpone or possibly prevent it. Fountain suggests that Americans are always worrying about the wrong illnesses, such as flesh-eating disease, a staph infection that affects maybe 1,500 Americans, or avian flu, which has yet to affect anyone in the United States, rather than chronic illnesses like diabetes, which can be dealt with in part through diet and exercise.[21] Peter M. Sandman, a risk-communication consultant, advises, "There's got to be something for them to do. If you want people to take diabetes and their health issues seriously, you have to give them an agenda of things to do to stay well such as a one-time action such as a blood sugar test and longer-term changes in habits such as dieting and exercise."[22] Wellness teams can offer a *things-to-do* agenda.

Wellness team *actions* can not only help prevent long-term illnesses such as diabetes but also can provide intervention for the fifth of American men and more than a third of American women who, as Fountain reports,[23] say they would like to lose at least twenty pounds, and not become like Marty, the title character in Paddy Chayefsky's 1955 play, who whines, "I'm just a fat little man, a fat ugly man," or English journalist William Leith, whose overweight condition makes him feel "lousy and repulsive."[24] Wellness teams can offer the future young Martys and Williams of the world an intervention agenda so they don't have to endure a life feeling lousy, repulsive, and ugly.

And wellness team *actions* can help level the playing field for middle- and lower-class children and teens by providing them with regular physical activity and nutrition and education for their parents. Regular physical activity should not have to be purchased but should come as an important part of the school-day experience for each and every student. Wealthy parents can buy opportunities for daily exercise for their overweight and obese children. As reporter Mireya Navarro suggests, with health statistics pointing at an increasingly obese population, the national preoccupation with weight is leading the affluent parents of teenagers and even younger children to sign them up at a health-club gym tailored to them, hire personal trainers that may cost $100 an hour, and schedule physical workouts as they do piano lessons.[25]

The International Health, Racquet and Sports Club Association says that children are the second-fastest-growing market for health clubs after baby boomers over the age of fifty-five. More than 4.6 million American children between the ages of six and seventeen hold memberships in health clubs.[26] Wellness teams can take action to make sure regular physical activity is provided to those who can't afford health club memberships, personal trainers, and scheduled workouts outside of school. They, too, need something to do and an agenda to stay well.

As nutrition educator Ann M. Evans suggests, educators need to let students know, "Your school cares about your health and well-being. Your school practices wellness. You, the students, are our message to the future and we're sending you forward with knowledge." Evans's advice to educators, and, I would add, to school wellness teams, is, "It's not for lack of information that the crisis in children's health is escalating. We need to put first things first. We know what we need to do."[27] Putting first things first means making sure our children and teens are provided with healthy food and drink and regular physical activity as well as academic opportunities. Nutrition/physical activity and academics need to be equal partners in an education process that enables young people to learn how to keep their lives in good order. Wellness teams can be an ongoing safeguard and voice to make sure the equal partnership between academics and nutrition/physical activity stays on course in a world pushing academic achievement and relegating wellness to a lower priority.

In conclusion, I argue that our mission as educators is to provide an arena of comfort and safety for overweight and obese teens and to let them know that their school cares about their health and well-being by offering many open doors to learn how to develop and maintain a healthy lifestyle. Indeed, we know what to do to answer the call of overweight teens like Fred Rogers, who became famous for his PBS Mr. Rogers role. Rogers's remarks put a real face on what it feels like to be an overweight teen on the run from bullying, searching for an arena of comfort and an open door for help, and finding it in the care and modeling of extraordinary and ordinary adults such as teachers and grandparents. Here are Rogers's memories of his teen years:

When I was a kid, I was shy and overweight. I was a perfect target for ridicule. One day (how well I remember that day, and it's more than sixty years ago!) we got out of school early, and I started to walk home by myself. It wasn't long before I sensed I was being followed— by a whole group of boys. As I walked faster, I looked around, and they started to call my name and came close and closer and got louder and louder, "Freddy, hey, fat Freddy. We are going to get you, fat Freddy." I resented those kids for not seeing beyond my fatness or my shyness. And I didn't know that it was all right to resent it, to feel bad about it, even to feel very sad. I didn't know it was all right to feel any of those things, because the advice I got from grown-ups was, "Just let on you don't care, then nobody will bother you." What I actually did was mourn. I cried to myself whenever I was alone. I cried through my fingers as I made up songs on the piano. I sought out stories of other people who were poor in spirit, and I felt for them.

I started to look behind the things that people did and said and little by little concluded that Saint-Exupery was absolutely right when he wrote in *The Little Prince*, "What is essential is invisible to the eye." So after a lot of sadness, I began a lifelong search for what is essential. I don't know how this came to me, maybe through one of my teachers or from my grandfather, who used to say to me after we had a visit together, "Freddy, you made this day a special day for me." My hunch is all those extraordinary, ordinary people who believed that I was more than I thought I was, all those saints who helped a fat, shy kid to see more clearly what was really essential.[28]

Wellness team members may not be saints, but they can educate, counsel, and encourage "fat" teens like Fred Rogers not to settle for a role in life that advises them to "let on you don't care, then nobody will bother you." Overweight and obese teens need to avoid sliding into a role of turning the other cheek and, as Rogers said so well, beginning to accept and live their lives feeling it all right to resent ridicule, to feel bad about it, even to feel sad about it, to mourn and cry to oneself. They must be offered encouragement and hope and a place in the school community with caring adults who believe, as in Rogers's case, "that I was more than I thought I was." They need adults who have the gift of being very aware of teens who are fat and shy and know what to do to help them become contributing members of the school community, not leave them on the outside looking in. That is not simply *intervention* but *loving intervention*, as was the case with the young Bill Fibkins being welcomed into the school community and shown how to contribute, to be in the club, by Bill Carmichael, Ervin Fieger, and Ward Donner.

NOTES

1. National Alliance for Nutrition and Activity (NANA), "Model Local School Wellness Policies on Physical Activity and Nutrition," Center for Science in the Public Interest, Mar. 2005, http://www.schoolwellnesspolicies.org (accessed 2 June 2005), 15.

2. The Center for Ecoliteracy, "Model Wellness Policy Guide," 1 Sept. 2005, http://www.ecoliteracy.org (accessed 3 Jan. 2006), 9–10.

3. American Diabetes Association, "Corporate Health Ambassador Case Study: Lisa Holland's Story," American Diabetes Association case study, 2005, http://www.diabetes.org/support-the-cause/corporate-friends/statefarm.jsp (accessed 24 May 2005).

4. American Diabetes Association, "Corporate Health Ambassador Case Study."

5. Wellness Councils of America (WELCOA), "Fitness Driven," WELCOA Expert Interview, 2005, http://www.welcoa.org (accessed 10 Jan. 2006).

6. Singapore Ministry of Health (MOH), "Ministry of Health Counts Steps Towards A Healthy Lifestyle," MOH press release, 19 May 2004, http://www2.coca-cola.com/presscenter/pc_include/nr_20040519_singapore_stepwithit (accessed 29 Nov. 2005).

7. Business Group Health, "Pitney Bowes: Obesity Initiative," 29 Nov. 2005, http://www.wgbh.com/healthy/pitneybowes_obesityinitiative.efm? (accessed 19 Nov. 2005).

8. Jennifer Hutchins, "Health Is Serious Business at Daimler-Chrysler Corporate Wellness Programs," LookSmart, 2005, http://www.findarticles.com/p/articles/mi_m0FXS/is_9_78/ai_65650783 (accessed 29 Nov. 2005).

9. Gina Bellafante, "The Governor Who Put His State on a Diet," *New York Times*, 10 Aug. 2005, F2.

10. Stephanie Sullivan (now Stephanie Sullivan Pittman, PHR), "Wellness Programs," healthresources.com, 2 Nov. 2000, http://www.e-hresources.com/Articles/Nov2.htm (accessed 29 Nov. 2005).

11. Malin Lundblad, "Corporate Wellness," *OC Metro*, 14 Apr. 2005, http://www.ocmetro.com/archives.ocmetro_2005.metro041405.health0414 05.html (accessed 29 Nov. 2005).

12. Sullivan, "Wellness Programs."

13. Sullivan, "Wellness Programs."

14. Sullivan, "Wellness Programs."

15. Sullivan, "Wellness Programs."

16. Sullivan, "Wellness Programs."

17. Sullivan, "Wellness Programs."

18. Sullivan, "Wellness Programs."

19. Sullivan, "Wellness Programs."

20. Radical HealthWorks, "Proposals in Support of a Nutrition Education Program in the Workplace," 2004, http://www.radicalhealthworks .com/nutrition.html (accessed 29 Nov. 2005).

21. Henry Fountain, "On Not Wanting to Know What Hurts You," *New York Times*, 15 Jan. 2006, Weekly section, 14.

22. Fountain, "On Not Wanting to Know," 14.

23. Fountain, "On Not Wanting to Know," 14.

24. Steven Shapin, "Eat and Run," *The New Yorker*, 16 January 2006, 76.

25. Mireya Navarro, "Playtime at the Health Club," *New York Times*, sec. 9, pp. 1, 10.

26. Navarro, "Playtime at the Health Club," sec. 9, pp. 1, 10.

27. Ann M. Evans, "What in Health Is Going on Here?" The Center for Ecoliteracy, 12 Jan. 2006, http://www.ecoliteracy.org/publications/rsl/ ann-evans.htm (accessed 12 Jan. 2006).

28. Fred Rogers, *Life's Journeys According to Mister Rogers* (New York: Hyperion, 2005), 18–21.